Cross Infection Control in Dentistry:
a practical illustrated guide

Peter R. Wood, BchD
Leeds
England

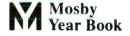
Mosby
Year Book

St. Louis   Baltimore   Boston   Chicago   London   Philadelphia   Sydney   Toronto

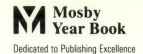

Mosby Year Book

Dedicated to Publishing Excellence

Contents

Preface

Cross infection control is an integral part of dentistry and many dental healthcare workers no longer question its necessity.

Universal cross infection control procedures are now implemented when treating each patient, following the inevitable realisation that a large majority of carriers of infectious diseases cannot be identified.

Such universal precautions must be both comprehensive, to prevent infection transmission in all clinical situations, and realistic, to allow convenient provision of dental treatment.

This book describes updated regulations, recommendations, and practical techniques, which it is hoped may enable dental healthcare workers to provide realistic, but safe, universal precautions for every patient.

Peter R. Wood
Leeds
England

Acknowledgements

My wife Ann has given support, encouragement, and practical help in typing the manuscript; first and foremost I thank her.

The support and advice provided by my good friend and colleague Dr Michael Martin has been invaluable, not only during the time preparing this book but also in the recent few years. It is very much appreciated.

I must thank Alwyne Gardner for producing such excellent clinical photographs and Ann, Pam, Lisa, and Vicki for help in producing these.

So many people have kindly provided help, material and information for the book. The following deserve special and equal thanks:

Professor James Crawford, University of North Carolina, USA
Dr Rella Christenson, Director, Clinical Research Associates, USA
Professor John Molinari, University of Detroit School of Dentistry, USA
Professor Bjorn Hurlen, University of Oslo, Norway
Professor John Young, University of Texas, USA
Professor Virginia Merchant, University of Detroit School of Dentistry, USA
Professor Mark Marener, Temple University School of Dentistry, USA
Professor Chrispian Scully, University of Bristol Dental School, UK
Dr Chris Miller, Indiana School of Dentistry, USA
Dr David Lamb, University of Sheffield, UK
Dr Ann Field, Liverpool School of Dentistry, UK
Dr Carolyn Gray, American Association of Dental Schools, Washington DC, USA
Professor Peter Rothwell, University of Sheffield, UK
Dr Colin Wall, Director, Australian Dental Association, Australia
Dr Karlheinz Kimmel, Director, International Institute of Dental Practice Administration, Germany
Dr John Edwards, St Marks Clinic, New Zealand
Ann Marie Regmery, International Dental Association, London, UK
Dr Jack Cooke, General Dental Practitioner, Leeds, UK
Margaret Clennett, British Dental Association Library, UK
Dr Dan Langen, Council on Dental Therapeutics, American Dental Association, USA
Dr Barbara Gooch, Centers for Disease Control, USA
Susan Hall Fleming, US Department of Labor, Washington DC, USA
David Phillips and Dental Protection Ltd, Medical Protection Society, UK
Dr Michael Baron, Brantford, USA
Kathy Bernard, Products Manager, Hu Friedy Ltd, USA
Derek Gee, Castellini UK Ltd, UK
Bruce Finnigen and Steven Lawry, Whaledent International, New York, USA
Andrew Carr, Eschmann Equipment Ltd, UK
Frederik Echert, Siemens, Germany
Jim Bohan, Antec International, UK
Brian Whitby, Adec, USA
Ray Allen, Dentronix Inc, Ivyland, USA
Thomas Stumpf, Cox Sterile Products Inc, USA
Diane Miller, The Hygenic Corporation, USA
Dr Ish Pankhania, 3M Health Care Ltd, UK
Dr David Rees, Dental Protection Society Ltd, UK
Dr L. Samaranayake, Prince Philip Dental Hospital, Hong Kong
Dr W.J. Cunliffe, Consultant Dermatologist, Leeds General Infirmary, UK
Dr D.M.G. Main, Department of Oral Medicine, Leeds Dental Hospital, UK

The following Dental Associations provided information and advice:

Barbados
Sweden
Netherlands
Israel
South Africa
Germany
France
Hong Kong
Australia
Norway
Kenya
New Zealand
Denmark
America
United Kingdom

Peter R. Wood
Leeds
England

Introduction

The future presents a myriad of concerns, regulations, and changing practice styles to all dental practitioners. Recently, two separate occurrences have reinforced these concerns.

The implications of the Occupational Safety and Health Administration (OSHA) guidelines have affected the way in which all dentists in the USA now practise. Dental offices with at least one employee must comply with the infection control requirements stated in the OSHA regulations. Good cross infection control, together with the maintenance of careful written records and instructions as prescribed by the OSHA rule, are now mandatory in the USA. Violations can result in fines levied by OSHA, but state and local regulations may have greater impact. The incorporation of OSHA regulations into municipal and state ordinances may result in suspension or revocation of a dentist's licence to practise if violation is found. The legal implications of recently introduced regulations may seem insurmountable to many practising dentists in the USA, but it is essential that they are familiar with and implement existing municipal state and federal regulations.

In many other countries new regulations are being introduced. The responsibility for cross infection control lies with the practising dentist who, in the 1990s and beyond, will have increasing responsibilities; the concerns of the dentists in the USA must be shared by dentists worldwide.

The second occurrence is of great concern to all dental healthcare workers worldwide. Recently, the Centers for Disease Control (CDC), Atlanta, reported several patients who became infected with human immunodeficiency virus (HIV) during treatment by the same HIV-infected dentist who practised in Florida. These patients and the dentist in question were infected with the same strain of HIV and this was distinct from strains collected at random from other HIV-infected individuals in the same community.

Dental healthcare workers must review procedures employed in their offices, to prevent the transmission of infection. Careful cross infection control as described in the relevant regulations and guidelines must be applied on every occasion that treatment is provided.

1. Transmission of Infection

It is essential that all dental healthcare workers have a basic understanding of infection transmission. This chapter summarises the factors that influence transmission and the risks involved.

Infection transmission during dental procedures is dependent on four factors (**1.1**).

---

1. Source of infection
The source of infection may be a patient or a member of the dental team who is suffering from, or is a carrier of, an infectious disease.

2. Means of transmission
Micro-organisms capable of causing disease are present in human blood. Contact with blood or saliva mixed with blood may transmit such pathogenic micro-organisms from one person to another. Pathogenic micro-organisms must be present over a certain concentration within blood or saliva to overcome the body's defences. This is known as the minimum infective dose.

3. Route of transmission
Transmission may occur by *inoculation* or *inhalation*:

- Previously damaged skin or mucous membrane provides a portal of entry for micro-organisms.
- Contaminated needles, sharp instruments, or flying debris from the oral cavity may penetrate the skin.
- Inhalation of contaminated aerosols is a possible route of transmission.

4. Susceptible host
A susceptible host is a person who lacks effective resistance to a particular pathogenic micro-organism. Many factors influence a person's level of susceptibility to a particular infectious agent. Heredity, nutritional status, medications such as steroids, therapeutic procedures such as chemotherapy, and underlying diseases such as diabetes, all increase the risk and the severity of infection. Immunisation status is also a factor that influences susceptibility.

1.1 Factors determining transmission of infection during dental procedures.

Source of Infection

The source of infection may be divided into *three* main groups (**1.2**).

1.2 Of the sources, patients who suffer from acute infections do not usually seek dental treatment; patients who seek dental treatment during the *prodromal stage* of an infection appear healthy but may be infectious; and the carriers of infectious diseases are divided into two sub-groups: (a) those who have suffered acute illness, recovered, and become carriers (members of this group are usually identified), and (b) those who unknowingly have a subclinical infection and go on to become carriers. This is the majority group, whose members *cannot usually be identified*, and is the **danger** group that is cause for concern.

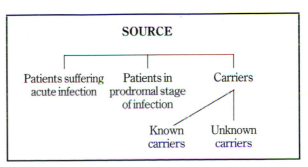

The risk of infection following exposure

Not all exposures result in infection. The risk of becoming infected by hepatitis B virus (HBV) and HIV, as well as other pathogens, is influenced by several factors, including:

- Route of exposure, e.g. parenteral exposure.
- Differences in host susceptibility.
- The dose of the virus transferred during an exposure incident.
- The number of exposure incidents.

For example, the risk of infection increases as the number of virus particles transferred during an exposure incident increases, and with increasing numbers of exposure incidents.

Infection control

The goal of infection control is to eliminate the transfer of micro-organisms. This may be accomplished in several ways:

- Use of personal barrier equipment.
- Proper techniques for handling sharp instruments.
- Immunisation of dental healthcare workers against infectious diseases of concern, and maintenance of general good health to decrease their susceptibility to infections.
- Correct cleaning and disinfection of surfaces and equipment to remove infectious agents.
- Sterilisation of instruments.

Risk to Dental Staff

Dentists, dental assistants, hygienists, laboratory technicians, secretarial staff, cleaning staff, and dental engineers are all at risk[1] from cross infection and must be protected. The risk is high, and in a dental practice that sees 20 patients a day, it has been estimated that in a one-week period an average of at least two patients with oral herpes, one hepatitis B carrier, and an unknown number of individuals with HIV will be encountered.[2]

Several studies[1,3-6] have attempted to define the risk to individual members of the dental team, and they suggest that members of the dental team have a higher risk than the general population of contracting infections.

How dental staff acquire infections

Injuries caused by contaminated instruments

Injuries caused by contaminated instruments may create a portal of entry for pathogenic micro-organisms. If the number of micro-organisms introduced by this route exceeds the infective dose, infection may result. It has been reported that the majority of dentists recall needlestick injuries over a period of 3 years, with an average of one needlestick per year.[7]

Risk of infection following needlestick injury
It has been estimated that the volume of blood in a needlestick injury is quite small (1.4 µl).[8] Prospective studies into the risk of contracting HIV infection from a needlestick injury all come to the same conclusion, that the risk of sero-conversion, after needlestick injury from an HIV-infected person, is about 0.4%.[9,10] At present, only one dentist who was not at increased risk of HIV infection from high-risk behaviour, has been reported as HIV positive.[10] Conversely, minute quantities of blood, estimated at only 0.1 µl, may be sufficient for parenteral transmission of hepatitis B. The combined data from prospective studies[11,12] indicate the risk of infection with HBV after a needlestick injury is 20–25%.

Injuries by contaminated instruments present a *major* risk to the dental team, and care must be taken at all times when handling needles and other sharp instruments.

Existing lesions on the operator's hands

The incidence of HBV infection among the dental profession is about five times higher than in the general population.[4–6,13] The most likely mode of transmission is via the operator's hands. It has been reported that dentists have been infected with syphilis and herpes simplex by their patients, when ungloved hands contacted oral lesions during dental procedures.[14,15]

If members of the dental team operate ungloved, contact with blood and saliva is inevitable, and if breaks in hand skin are present these may serve as portals of entry for pathogenic micro-organisms. Allen and Organ[16] studied the presence of blood remnants on the fingers of dentists. Blood was found on 80% of the dentists examined, particularly under the nails and on the thumb and index finger. In 40% of cases, blood was still found on these areas after the weekend. The same study revealed microlesions in the hand skin of 40% of the dentists studied.

Members of the dental team who operate ungloved are at risk. Operating gloves should be worn during all dental procedures to protect the hands.

Dental aerosol

Dental aerosol is generated by turbine handpieces, air/water syringes, and ultrasonic scalers. Aerosol is defined as small droplets, usually 5 μm or less in diameter, which can remain suspended in air for some time. There is limited evidence that dental aerosols transmit infection to dental staff, but it has been found that respiratory-tract infections occur more frequently among dentists than among the general population.[17,18] *Mycobacterium tuberculosis* has been detected in dental aerosols[19] and studies have shown an increased incidence of tuberculosis in dental professionals.[20]

The spread of infection by dental aerosol is regarded as low risk. However, dentists, hygienists, and dental assistants are advised to wear a good-quality operating mask when providing dental treatment. Good ventilation, bacteriocidal pre-treatment mouth washes, electrostatic precipitation units, and high-speed vacuum aspiration reduce the level of contaminated aerosols.

Splashes of contaminated sharp material

When operating the turbine handpiece, particles over 0.1 mm in diameter are dispersed up to 6 m at speeds of 50–60 km/h. The dentist and dental assistant may sustain microtrauma to the eyes, face, and hands.[21–23] Such microlesions may serve as portals of entry for pathogenic micro-organisms contained in blood and saliva splashes generated during dental treatment. It has been suggested that hepatitis B and herpes simplex type I (manifesting as herpetic keratitis) are transmitted in this way.

The risks involved are moderate, but precautions should be taken using:

- Protective eye wear.
- Masks.

Risk to the Patient

There are few reports that describe transmission of diseases to the patient during dental treatment. This does not indicate that disease transmission to patients is low, but emphasises the difficulty in proving that cross infection to patients occurs during dental treatment. It has been reported that hepatitis B[24,25], syphilis[26], herpes simplex type I[26], tuberculosis[27], and micro-organisms causing oral abscesses[28–30] have been transmitted to patients during dental treatment.

The possible routes of transmission of infection to patients are summarised in **1.3**. The majority of cases of transmission from dental staff to patients occur via the hands.

1.3

1. Lesion on the operator's ungloved hand.
2. Contaminated operator's ungloved hands.
3. Contaminated instruments or other dental equipment.

1.3 Possible routes of transmission of infection to patients.

Surface contamination

During dental procedures, flying debris, aerosols, droplet splatter, and contaminated hands and instruments cause widespread contamination of the operating area.[31,32]

The possibility of transmission of infections by environmental surfaces continues to be questioned by some authorities. However, it has been shown that many pathogenic micro-organisms can survive on a variety of surfaces[33], which has given credibility to infection via contaminated surfaces. Studies have shown[34,35] that Rotavirus and Rhinovirus can be transferred from contaminated hands in sufficient numbers to cause infection in susceptible hosts. Colds caused by Rhinovirus have been transferred experimentally to human volunteers via contaminated cup handles.[36] At the clinical level, it is difficult to establish such transfer, and clinical reports linking infection with objects have been based on circumstantial evidence.[37] However, such reports make it impossible to rule out environmental surfaces as fomites.

References

[1]Underhill, T. E. and Terezhalmy, G. T. Epidemiologic aspects of infectious diseases important to dentists. *Comp. Cont. Ed. Dent.*, 1986;**7**:48–57.

[2]Crawford, J. State of the art practical infection control in dentistry. *J. Am. Dent. Assoc.*, 1985;**110**:629–33.

[3]Cottone, J. A. Hepatitis B virus infection in the dental profession. *J. Am. Dent. Assoc.* 1985;**110**:617–21.

[4]Feldman, R. E. and Schiff, E. R. Hepatitis in dental professionals. *JAMA,* 1975;**232**:1228–30.

[5]Mori, M. Status of viral hepatitis in the world community: its incidence among dentists and other dental personnel. *Int. Dent. J.*, 1984;**34**:115–21.

[6]Smith, J. L., Maynard, J. E., Berquist, K. R. *et al.* Comparative risk of hepatitis B among physicians and dentists. *J. Infect. Dis.*, 1976;**133**:705–6.

[7]Samaranayake, L. P., Lamey, P. J., MacFarlane, T. W., Glass, G. W. J. Attitudes of general dental practitioners towards the hepatitis B vaccine. *Community Dent. Oral Epidemiol.*, 1987;**15**:125–7.

[8]Napoli, V. M. and McGowan, J. E. How much blood is in a needlestick? *J. Infect. Dis.*, 1987;**155**:828.

[9]Klein, R. S., Phelan, J. A., Freeman, K. *et al.* Low occupational risk of HIV infection among dental professionals. *N. Engl. J. Med.*, 1988;**318**:86–90.

[10]Centers for Disease Control. Acquired immunodeficiency syndrome and human immunodeficiency virus infection among healthcare workers. *Morb. Mort. Weekly Report*, 1988;**37**:229–34.

[11]Barker, L. J. Transmission of serum Hepatitis. *JAMA,* 1970;**211**:1509–12.

[12]Grady, G. F., Lee, V.A., Prince, A. M. *et al.* Hepatitis B immune globulin for accidental exposure among medical personnel: final report of a multicentre controlled trial. *J. Infect. Dis.*, 1978;**138**:625–8.

[13]American Association of Public Health Dentistry. (Annual Meeting, 30 October – 1 November 1985.) The control of transmissible diseases in dental practice. A position paper of the American Association of Public Health Dentistry. *J. Public Health Dent.*, 1986;**46**:13–21.

[14]Brooks, S. L., Rowe, N. H., Drach, J. C. *et al.* Prevalence of the herpes simplex virus disease in a professional population. *J. Am. Dent. Assoc.*, 1981;**102**: 31–4.

[15]Rowe, N. H., Heine, C. S., Kowalski, C. J. Herpetic whitlow: an occupational disease of practising dentists. *J. Am. Dent. Assoc.*, 1982;**105**:471–3.

[16]Allen, A. L. and Organ, R. J. Occult blood under the fingernails: a mechanism for the spread of blood-borne infection. *J. Am. Dent. Assoc.*, 1982;**105**:455–9.

[17]Rosen, S., Schmakel, D., Schoener, M. Incidence of respiratory disease in dental hygienists and dieticians. *Clin. Prev. Dent.*, 1985;**7**:24–5.

[18]Rowe, N. H. and Brooks, S. L. Contagion in the dental office. *Dent. Clin. North Am.*, 1978;**22**:491–503.

[19]Belting, C. M., Haberford, G. C., Juhl, L. K. Spread of organisms from dental air rotor. *J. Am. Dent. Assoc.*, 1964;**68**:34–47.

[20]Shaw, B. A. Tuberculosis in medical and dental students. *Lancet*, 1952;**2**:400–4.

[21]Hartley, J. L. Eye and face injuries resulting from dental procedures. *Dent. Clin. North Am.*, 1978;**22**:505–16.

[22]Grandy, J. R. Enamel aerosols created during use of the air turbine handpiece. *J. Dent. Res.*, 1967;**46**:409–16.

[23]Kramer, R. von. The dentist's health; high speed rotary equipment as a risk factor. *Quint. Internat.*, 1985;**16**: 367–71.

[24]Centers for Disease Control. Hepatitis B among dental patients. Indiana. *Morb. Mort. Weekly Report*, 1985; **34**:73–5.

[25]Kane, M. A. and Lettau, L. A. Transmission of HBV from the dental personnel to patients. *J. Am. Dent. Assoc.*, 1985;**110**:634–6.

[26]Manzella, J. P., McConville, J. H., Wiliam, V. *et al.* An outbreak of herpes simplex in a dental hygiene practice. *JAMA*, 1984;**252**:2019–22.

[27]Smith, W.H.R., Davies, D., Mason, K. D. et al. Intraoral and pulmonary tuberculosis following dental treatment. *Lancet*, 1982;**10**:842–4.

[28]Martin, M. V. The significance of the bacterial contamination of dental unit water systems. *Br. Dent. J.*, 1987;**163**: 152–4.

[29]Martin, M. V. and Hardy, P. Two cases of oral infection by methicillin resistant *Staphylococcus aureus*. *Br. Dent. J.*, 1991;**170**:63–5.

[30]Autio, K. L., Rosen, S., Reynolds, N. J., Bright, J. S.

Studies in cross contamination in the dental clinic. *J. Am. Dent. Assoc.*, 1980;**100**:358–61.

[31]Crawford, J. J. *If Saliva were Red.* 35 mm slide demonstration, Chapel Hill: University of North Carolina Dental School, 1979.

[32]Molinari, J. A. and York, J. Cross contamination visualisation. *JCDA*, 1987;**15**(9):12–16.

[33]Thomas, L. E., Sydiskis, R. J., de Vore, D. T., Krywolap, G. N. Survival of herpes simplex virus and other selected micro-organisms on patients' charts. Potential source of infection. *J. Am. Dent. Assoc.*, 1985;**111**:461–4.

[34]Pancic, F., Carpentier, D. C., Caine, P. E. Role of infectious secretions in the transmission of rhinovirus. *J. Clin. Microbiol.*, 1980;**12**:567–71.

[35]Ansari, S. A., Sattar, S. A., Springthorpe, V. S. *et al.* Survival on human hands and transfer of infectious virus to animate and nonporous inanimate surfaces. *J. Clin. Microbiol.*, 1988;**26**:1513–18.

[36]Gwaltney, J. M. Jr. and Hendley, J. O. Transmission of experimental rhinovirus infection by contaminated surfaces. *Am. J. Epidemiol.*, 1982;**116**:828–33.

[37]Christenson, R. P., Robinson, R. A., Robinson, D. F. *et al.* Antimicrobial activity of environmental surface disinfectants in the absence and presence of bioburden. *J. Am. Dent. Assoc.*, 1989;**119**:493–505.

2. Infections of Concern in Dentistry

This chapter describes infections which, evidence suggests, may be transmitted during dental procedures. Diseases transmitted by inoculation and inhalation are summarised in **Tables 2.1** and **2.2**.

Table 2.1 Micro-organisms transmitted by inoculation.

Micro-organism	Disease
Hepatitis B virus (HBV)	Hepatitis B
Hepatitis C virus (HCV)	Non-A, non-B, hepatitis
Hepatitis D virus (HDV)	Delta hepatitis
Herpes simplex type I	Oral herpes, herpetic whitlow, herpetic keratitis
Herpes simplex type II	Genital herpes
Human Immunodeficiency virus (HIV)	Acquired immunodeficiency syndrome (AIDS), AIDS-related complex (ARC)
Neisseria gonorrhoeae	Gonorrhoea
Treponema pallidum	Syphilis
Pseudomonas aeruginosa	Wound infections, abscesses
Staphylococcus aureus/ S. albus	Wound infections, abscesses
Clostridium tetani	Tetanus

Table 2.2 Micro-organisms transmitted by inhalation.

Micro-organism	Disease
Varicella virus	Chickenpox
Cytomegalovirus	Infection in infants
Measles (rubeola) and mumps viruses	Measles/mumps
Influenza virus Rhinovirus Adenovirus	Influenza and common cold
Rubella virus	German measles
Mycobacterium tuberculosis	Tuberculosis
Streptococcus pyogenes	Oral abscesses, rheumatic fever and endocarditis
Candida albicans	(Opportunistic) candidosis

A more detailed summary of infectious hazards may be found in the *Journal of the American Dental Association* report, 1988.[1]

To facilitate a better understanding of infection control, members of the dental team should possess a knowledge of infection transmission and of diseases that are of concern in dentistry.

A basic knowledge of the diseases covered in this chapter is essential.

AIDS and HIV Infection

There has been a dramatic increase in cases of AIDS and carriers of the human immunodeficiency virus (HIV). It is inevitable that increasing numbers of HIV carriers will attend dental surgeries. The majority of these carriers will be unidentified.

Progress of the disease

There are a number of possible sequelae once HIV enters the body.[2]

- The virus may stimulate antibody production. The incubation period for antibody production is 2–12 weeks. Early infection can produce a mild influenza type of illness with fever and sore throat, but then the patient may become asymptomatic.

- The virus may be incorporated into the nucleo-protein of T4 lymphocytes and carried in *latent* form for many years. About 90% of the total number of persons infected with HIV belong in this group, and may be unaware of their condition.[3] Unknown carriers of HIV are infectious, and it is generally believed that any patient seropositive for HIV anti-bodies remains infected and infectious for life.[4] Such a large undiagnosed group of infectious persons, which is rapidly increasing in numbers, ensures that the dental team will come into contact with unknown HIV carriers on a regular basis.

- The virus can be activated to reproduce itself and infect more lymphocytes.

- The virus depresses the number of T4 lympho-cytes, reducing the patient's immunity. The majority of the clinical signs and symptoms of the AIDS-related complex (ARC) and AIDS are a consequence of the patient's lack of immunity.

Risk groups

Homosexual men and intravenous drug users represent the largest groups of HIV-positive individuals. However, the proportion of heterosexual males and females who have acquired HIV infection is rapidly increasing and is cause for concern. Minority groups of HIV-positive individuals include recipients of un-screened blood transfusions and children born to HIV-positive mothers.

The human immunodeficiency virus

The virus is found in most body fluids. Semen and blood containing infected lymphocytes, are the main modes of transmission.[2] The concentration of HIV in saliva is low,[5] and saliva has been found to destroy the virus.[6]

HIV is easily destroyed outside the body, and normal disinfection and sterilisation techniques employed in routine cross infection control will prevent transmission of HIV. However, it has been found to survive for up to seven days in blood at room temperature.[7] This reinforces the case for strict cross infection control.

Risk of transmission

The risk of transmission during the provision of healthcare is low.[8] To date, the scientific literature has reported 26 cases of HIV-infected healthcare workers (including that of one dentist), with no reported non-occupational risk.[9] Reports describing possible transmission of HIV to several patients from an HIV-infected dentist[10] have caused considerable concern.

Oral manifestations of HIV

The oral signs and symptoms of HIV infection are often the first recognisable features of the disease.[11] The dentist is in a unique position to recognise soft-tissue lesions associated with HIV infection during routine dental examinations. The recognition of such changes is important for planning management and treatment. In addition, the dentist may play a significant role in arranging counselling, proper referral, and behaviour modification, which are so important for effective treatment and control.[11]

Oral candidosis

Acute pseudomembranous candidosis (oral thrush) is a common HIV-related oral infection. Other causes must be eliminated before a definitive diagnosis of HIV infection is reached. It presents as white or creamy plaques, usually on the soft palate, pharynx, and tongue (**2.1, 2.2**). The plaques can be removed, revealing a bleeding subepithelial surface.[11]

Chronic hyperplastic candidosis is an *occasional* feature of HIV infection. Unlike thrush, this lesion does not wipe off.

Erythematous candidosis presents as a red area without removable plaques. It is often located on the palate, dorsum of the tongue, and buccal mucosa.

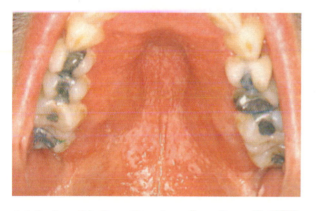

2.1 Oral candidosis on the palate of a patient with AIDS. (Courtesy Dr C.F. Farthing.)

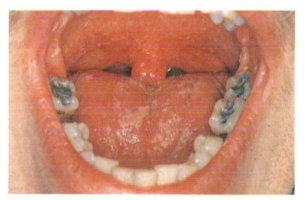

2.2

2.2 Oral candidosis on the tongue of a patient with AIDS. (Courtesy Dr C.F. Farthing.)

Hairy leukoplakia

Oral hairy leukoplakia is a lesion found predominantly on the lateral margins of the tongue (**2.3**).[11] It is usually white and does *not* rub off. It is seldom symptomatic. It is a significant clinical marker of HIV infection.[12]

Hairy leukoplakia is usually associated with the Epstein–Barr virus (EB virus). It is also occasionally found in immunocompromised individuals, such as post-operatively in renal, cardiac, or bone-marrow transplantation patients.

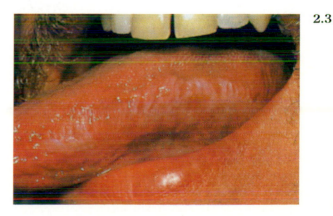

2.3

2.3 Hairy leukoplakia on the tongue. Note the distinctive ribbed appearance. (Courtesy Dr C.F. Farthing.)

Kaposi's sarcoma

Kaposi's sarcoma is a multicentre neoplasm of the vascular epithelium. Frequently, the first lesions appear in the mouth.[13] They can be red, blue, or purple and may be flat or raised, solitary or multiple.[11] It is commonly found on the hard palate (**2.4**), lesions starting adjacent to the second upper molar. Other sites include the gingivae (**2.5**), soft palate, and buccal mucosa.

2.4

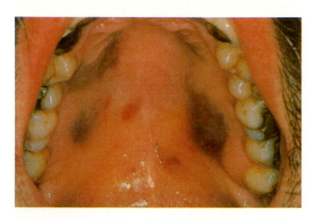

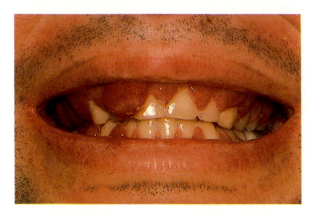

2.4   Kaposi's sarcoma lesions on the palate. (Courtesy Dr C.F. Farthing.)

2.5   Kaposi's sarcoma of the gingivae. (Courtesy C.F. Farthing.)

Herpes simplex virus and varicella virus

2.6

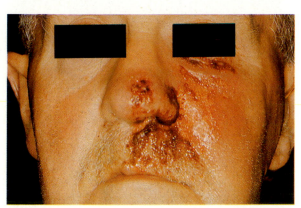

Herpes simplex type I can occasionally produce recurrent episodes of painful ulceration. The most common site is the lip, but lesions may occur in other areas, such as the gingivae, the palate, and the tongue.[11] Ulceration is typical of herpes simplex type I, but atypical forms may occur, including dendritic ulceration of the tongue. Herpes zoster infection (**2.6**) is a less common oral feature of HIV infection and is extremely painful.[14]

2.6   Herpes zoster infection. (Courtesy Dr Main.)

Gingivitis and periodontal disease

HIV-associated gingivitis (HIV-G) is an erythematous reaction of the gingivae, and may be prolonged and severe. It may progress to an acute necrotising ulcerative gingivitis (ANUG) (**2.7**).

HIV-associated periodontitis (HIV-P) presents as a rapid and irregular progressive destruction of the supporting tissues, the periodontal ligament, and the alveolar bone, with loosening of the teeth.[11] HIV-P may cause severe pain.

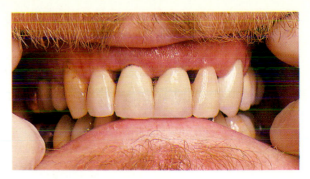

2.7 Necrotising ulcerative gingivitis in a patient with AIDS. (Courtesy Dr C.F. Farthing.)

Oral ulceration

The ulcers resemble aphthous ulceration (**2.8**), they are very painful, and may persist for several weeks.[11]

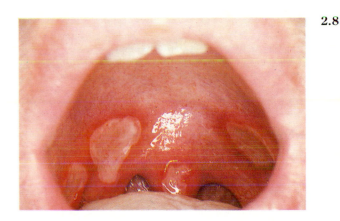

2.8 Aphthous ulcerations of the palate in a patient with AIDS. (Courtesy C.F. Farthing.)

Revised classification of HIV-associated oral lesions

In 1990, a working party composed of leading world authorities in oral medicine defined the clinical diagnostic criteria of lesions associated with HIV infection. These are shown in **Table 2.3**.

Table 2.3   Revised classification of HIV-associated oral lesions.

Group 1: Lesions strongly associated with HIV infection

Candidosis
   Erythematous
   Hyperplastic
   Pseudomembranous
Hairy leukoplakia (Epstein–Barr virus)
HIV gingivitis
Necrotising ulcerative gingivitis
HIV periodontitis
Kaposi's sarcoma
Non-Hodgkin's lymphoma

Group 2: Lesions less commonly associated with HIV infection

Atypical ulceration (oropharyngeal)
Idiopathic thrombocytopenic purpura
Salivary gland diseases
Viral infections other than Epstein–Barr virus:
   Cytomegalovirus
   Herpes simplex I virus
   Human papillomavirus (wart-like lesions)
   Varicella/H. zoster virus

Group 3: Lesions possibly associated with HIV infection

Hepatitis B

Hepatitis B is a major cause worldwide of acute and chronic hepatitis, cirrhosis, and primary hepatocellular carcinoma.

Hepatitis B remains a problem, and its prevalence appears to be increasing. There are over 200 million HBV carriers in the world[15], one million of them in the USA. In the USA, approximately 12,000 healthcare workers a year become infected with the virus. The Centers for Disease Control (CDC) have estimated that HBV infection in healthcare workers results in approximately 600 hospitalisations and 250 deaths each year in the USA.

HBV is a heat-resistant virus, destroyed after 5 minutes at 95°C.[16] The virus may survive for up to a week on work surfaces, and for longer than this on contaminated instruments.[17]

HBV is found in blood and blood products, i.e. saliva, sputum, breast milk, tears, wound fluid, sperm, sweat, urine, and vaginal discharges. Minute quantities of fluid may be sufficient for parenteral transmission (e.g. 0.1 μl of blood).[16]

Transmission of HBV

Percutaneous inoculation
This can occur either through contaminated needles and other instruments[18], or through microscopic skin lesions, i.e. cuticle lesions, eczema, or microtrauma caused by fast-moving airborne particles.[19]

Non-percutaneous infection via intact barriers
This occurs when contaminated tissue fluids come into contact with intact mucous membranes of oral and nasal mucosa.[18]

Indirect transmission
The environment must be regarded as contaminated after treatment of an HBV-positive patient, since HBV is very stable outside the body.[20]

Transmission during dental procedures

There is ample evidence supporting the transmission of hepatitis B from patients to dental staff and, less commonly, from dental staff to patients.[21,22]

Due to immunisation, the risk of dental staff contracting HBV is falling. Only half those infected with HBV have a clinically diagnosed illness, therefore 50% cannot give a history of illness. Of this group, 10% become carriers for one year and 5% carriers for several years.[23] The incubation period may be up to six months. The progress of the disease is illustrated in **2.9**.

The groups at risk for hepatitis B are[24]:

- Drug addicts (intravenous).
- Male homosexuals and bisexuals.
- Patients living in institutions.
- Patients who have spent their lives in developing countries.
- Patients with acute or chronic liver disease.
- Recipients of unscreened blood or blood products.
- Healthcare personnel.
- Oncology and dialysis patients.

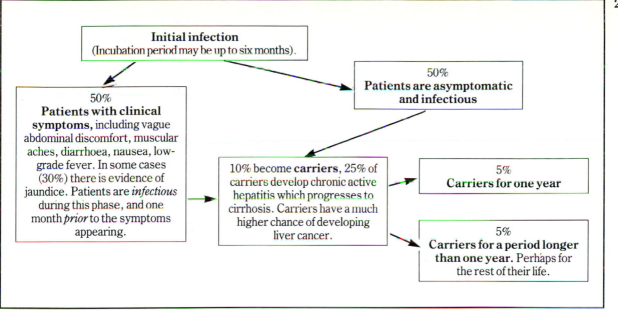

2.9   Progress of hepatitis B infection.

Summary

Hepatitis B is a cause for concern to all members of the dental team.

- There is widespread incidence of hepatitis B.
- A chronic carrier state is common.
- The virus survives well outside the body both on instruments and on surfaces, and is relatively resistant to disinfectants.
- Minute amounts of body fluids can transmit infection.

Dentists must be vaccinated against hepatitis B, and must ensure that all members of the dental team who are involved in clinical procedures are also vaccinated.

Delta Hepatitis – Hepatitis D

The delta hepatitis virus (HDV) is a defective-RNA virus, dependent on HBV for replication and transmission.[25] Hepatitis D is endemic in southern Italy and has been detected worldwide.[26] The disease is becoming more prevalent in the USA, especially in intravenous drug abusers, and several outbreaks have occurred. Groups at risk for Hepatitis D infection are[27]:

- **Asymptomatic hepatitis B surface antigen (HBsAg) carriers:**

Intravenous drug abusers
Haemodialysis patients
Male homosexuals who are also drug abusers
Institutionalised persons
Healthcare workers with frequent blood exposure.

- **Patients with liver disease:**
Acute hepatitis B
Chronic hepatitis B

Transmission of HDV

HDV infection takes place only in the presence of HBV, either in combination with acute HBV infection, or as a superinfection in a chronic HBV carrier. If a delta agent causes acute hepatitis, it may precipitate fulminant liver disease.

Hepatitis D is a serious threat to all members of the dental team. Transmission occurs in the same way as hepatitis B. If any one of the team (dentist, dental hygienist, dental assistant, or dental laboratory assistant) is a positive carrier of hepatitis D, then he or she may transmit both hepatitis B *and* hepatitis D to other individuals.[25] The vaccine currently available against hepatitis B infection will also prevent hepatitis D transmission.

Non-A Non-B Hepatitis

Non-A non-B hepatitis is caused by several viruses, including the virus responsible for hepatitis C infection.[28]

Hepatitis C infection is transmitted by blood and by blood products. The vaccine against hepatitis B infection does not provide protection against hepatitis C.

Hepatitis C infection is transmitted either enterically or parenterally. After infection with the hepatitis C virus, most people have subclinical infections, but the most significant known long-term consequence of parenteral hepatitis C is the high frequency of chronic liver disease.[28]

The risk of transmission of hepatitis C infection during routine dental practice is not clear.[28] At present there is no evidence of transmission, but, as the virus has been found in saliva, the possibility of transmission cannot be excluded.

Cytomegalovirus

Cytomegalovirus (CMV) has been identified as a source of infection in newborn infants. The number of carriers of this disease is increasing. CMV has received little attention, but in the USA it is a major cause of birth defects due to an infectious agent. The prenatal infection causes congenital hearing problems and mental retardation by attacking the central nervous system.

CMV survives on dried surfaces for long periods; it is shed in the saliva and possibly transmitted during dental procedures.[29] Pregnant women who work in close contact with patients, especially young children of preschool age, must be protected. Many commercial laboratories employ young women of childbearing age. Good cross infection control is essential because of the potential of CMV to survive on dental impressions and prosthetic and orthodontic appliances.

Tuberculosis

The increasing incidence of tuberculosis (TB), which began in 1986, is a cause for concern in the USA. There are two reasons for this increase: firstly, the increasing number of immigrants from countries which have a high incidence of TB infection; and secondly, persons infected with HIV may exhibit a comparatively high rate of secondary TB infection.

Mycobacterium tuberculosis is present in sputum, and disseminations of TB by aerosol formation (coughing) are common. Unvaccinated members of the dental team treating a patient with open TB are at risk of contracting the disease, if good cross infection control is not practised.[30] It is advisable for healthcare workers to be vaccinated against TB.

Syphilis

Syphilis is a four-stage disease following infection with *Treponema palidium*. The multiform skin eruptions of secondary syphilis and the hard chancre of primary syphilis may be sources of infection. Oral manifestations of this disease are frequently overlooked. Transmission of the disease may occur by contact with infected blood. Syphilis is common amongst AIDS patients.

T. palidium cannot survive for long periods outside the body and is easily destroyed by disinfection and by cooling. The dental team are at risk through contact with the skin and with the mucosal lesions of primary and secondary syphilis in and around the oral cavity.[31]

Transmission may occur through microlesions on the hands of members of the dental team who operate ungloved.[31]

Herpes Simplex Type I

This is the most common viral infection after the common cold and influenza. It is estimated that 50% of persons in the USA suffer from re-activated herpes simplex type I.[32]

Primary herpes simplex I

Primary acute gingivostomatitis is the first manifestation of this disease. Small, red, vesicular lesions are located on the palate, buccal mucosa and lips. These may coalesce to form large ulcerations. Other signs and symptoms may include enlarged lymph nodes, malaise, and gingival involvement (**2.10**). The acute phase lasts up to 14 days and occurs mainly in children aged 3–6 years, but it is now seen occasionally in adults.

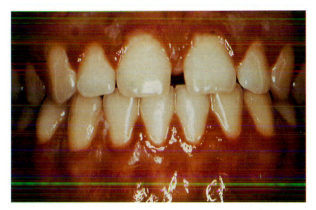

2.10

2.10 Primary acute gingivostomatitis. (Courtesy Dr M. V. Martin.)

Recurrent herpes simplex

After the initial infection, the virus (HSV-I) is harboured in the neural ganglion and may be re-activated by factors such as stress, ultraviolet light, allergy, menstrual cycle, and fatigue. After re-activation, small localised vesicles (cold sores) form on the lips (**2.11**), palate or buccal oral mucosa. These are similar to the lesions seen in the primary infection. Prior to the formation of herpetic lesions there may be an itching or burning sensation of the affected oral tissues.

The virus is relatively stable, especially in the presence of proteins (blood, saliva, etc.). It may survive for up to 4 hours at room temperature[33], but is both heat and acid sensitive and is easily destroyed by disinfectants.

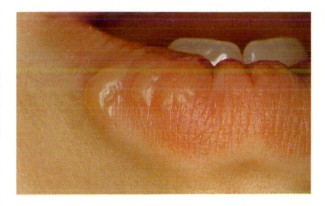

2.11

2.11 Secondary herpes simplex infection of the lip. (Courtesy Dr Main.)

Transmission

The disease may be transmitted from dental healthcare workers to patients[34], and from patients to dental healthcare workers. Infection may be transmitted to the non-immune dental operator: by unprotected hand contact with vesicle fluid, from primary or secondary lesions; by transfer of the vesicle fluid by rubbing of the eyes; or through eye injuries caused by contaminated dental splatter. It is essential that operating gloves and eye protection are worn when treating patients who are in the primary or recurrent stages of herpes simplex I infection. If possible, treatment of patients in the acute stages of this highly infectious disease should be postponed.

Manifestation in dental healthcare workers

Herpetic whitlow

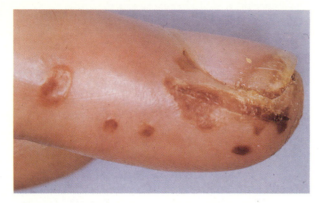

2.12   Herpetic whitlow. (Courtesy Dr M. V. Martin.)

It has been reported that dentists have been infected with herpes simplex I when their ungloved hands contacted oral lesions during dental procedures.[35] The herpetic whitlow found on the fingertip around the nail bed (**2.12**) may persist for several weeks, resulting in considerable inconvenience to the dental healthcare worker. The incubation period is 2–12 days, followed by an intense tingling in the operator's finger and a severe throbbing pain. The area involved is red and swollen. Vesicles erupt which may ulcerate and coalesce. New satellite vesicles may appear. Fever, chills, and malaise may accompany the first signs and symptoms.

It is essential that dental healthcare workers wear operating gloves, as microlesions have been found in the hand skin of 40% of dentists.[36] Occupational infection is fortunately now uncommon.

Herpetic keratitis

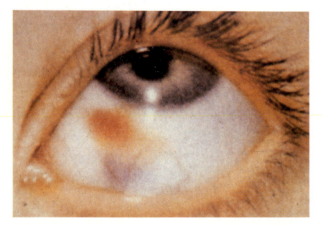

2.13   Herpetic keratitis. (Courtesy Dr M. V. Martin.)

Eye injuries caused by contaminated flying particles generated while using the turbine handpiece, the ultrasonic scaler, and the air/water syringe, may cause considerable inconvenience. Transmission of herpes simplex I may occur either by eye contact with flying particles, or following eye contact with the operator's contaminated hands. Herpetic keratitis (**2.13**) may cause permanent eye damage.

Primary herpetic stomatitis

Herpes simplex type I infection may be transferred from a patient to the healthcare worker, who may develop the clinical signs and symptoms of primary herpetic stomatitis.

Transmission of herpes simplex I may be prevented by wearing latex operating gloves and protective eyewear.

References

[1] American Dental Association Research Institute. Infectious hazards for both dental personnel and patients in the operatory. *J. Am. Dent. Assoc.*, 1988;**117**: 474–83.

[2] Silverman, S. Jr. Infectious disease control and the dental office: AIDS and other transmissible diseases. *Int. Dent. J.*, 1987;**87**:108–13.

[3] Barr, C. E. and Marder, M. Z. *AIDS, a Guide for Dental Practice*. Chicago Quintessence International Co. Inc., 1987.

[4] Farthing, C. F., Brown, S. E., Straughton, R. C. *A Colour Atlas of AIDS*, 2nd edn. Wolfe Medical Publications Ltd., London, 1988.

[5] Ho, D. D., Byington, R. E., Schooley, R. T., Flynn, R. T., Rota, T. R., Hirsh, M. S. Infrequency of isolation of HTLV III virus from saliva in AIDS. *N. Engl. J. Med.*, 1985;**313**:1606.

[6] Fox, P. C., Wolff, A., Yeh, C.-K. *et al.* Saliva inhibits HIV infectivity. *J. Am. Dent. Assoc.*, 1988;**116**:635–7.

[7] Resnick, L., Veren, K., Salahuddin, S., Tondreau, S., Markham, P. D. Stability and inactivation of HTLV–III/LAV under clinical and laboratory environments. *JAMA*, 1986;**255**:188–9.

[8] Scully, C. The level of risk of transmission of human immunodeficiency virus between patients and dental staff. *Br. Dent. J.*, 1991;**170**:97–100.

[9] Samaranayake, L. The risk of HIV transmission in dentistry. *Dental Update*, 1990;**17(6)**: 241–3.

[10] Centers for Disease Control. Possible transmission of human immunodeficiency virus to a patient during an invasive dental procedure. *Morb. Mort. Weekly Report*, 1990; **39**:448–93. Update: Transmission of HIV infection during an invasive dental procedure – Florida. *Morb. Mort. Weekly Report*, 1991;**40**:22–3.

[11] Greenspan, D. and Greenspan, J. S. The oral clinical features of HIV infection. *Gast. Clin. N. Am.*, 1988; **17**:535–43.

[12] Greenspan, D., Greenspan, J. S., Hearst, N. Relation of oral hairy leucoplakia to infection with HIV and the risk of developing AIDS. *J. Infect. Dis.*, 1987;**155**:475.

[13] Keeney, K., Albaza, D., Tidwell, D. *et al.* Oral Kaposi's sarcoma in acquired immune deficiency syndrome. *J. Oral Maxillofac. Surg.*, 1987;**45**:815–21.

[14] Ogden, G. R. and Chisholm, D. M. Orofacial manifestations of AIDS. *Dental Update*, 1988;**15**(10):420–3.

[15] Holliger, F. B. and Melnick, J. L. Overview. In: Holliger, Melnick, and Robinson (Eds.) *Viral Hepatitis*. pp. 1–6, New York, Raven Press, 1985.

[16] Barker, L. J. Transmission of serum hepatitis. *JAMA*, 1970;**211**:1509–12.

[17] Bond, W. W., Favaro, M. S., Peterson, N. J. *et al.* Survival of hepatitis B virus after drying and storage for one week. *Lancet*, 1981;**1**:550–1.

[18] Mosley, J. W. Present knowledge of viral hepatitis. *Int. Dent. J.*, 1984;**4**:110–14.

[19] Hartley, J. L. Eye and face injuries resulting from dental procedures. *Dent. Clin. N. Am.*, 1978;**22**:505–16.

[20] Favaro, M. S. Detection methods by study of the stability of the hepatitis B antigen on surfaces. *Infect. Dis.*, 1974; **129**:210–12.

[21] Centers for Disease Control. Hepatitis B among dental patients. Indiana. *Morb. Mort. Weekly Report*, 1985;**34**: 73–5.

[22] Kane, M. A. and Lettau, L. A. Transmission of HBV from dental personnel to patients. *J. Am. Dent. Assoc.*, 1985; **110**:634–6.

[23] Cottone, J. Hepatitis and the dental profession. *J. Am. Dent. Assoc.*, 1985;**110**:617–21.

[24] Ross, J. and Clarke, S. K. Hepatitis B in dentistry: the current position. *Br. Dent. J.*, 1981;**150**:89–91.

[25] Cottone, J. Delta hepatitis: another concern for dentistry. *J. Am. Dent. Assoc.*, 1986;**112**:47–9.

[26] Rizzeto, M. The Delta Agent, *Hepatology*, 1983;**3**:729–37.

[27] Centers for Disease Control. ACIP recommendations for protection against viral hepatitis. *Morb. Mort. Weekly Report*, 1985;**34**:313–35.

[28] Porter, S. R. and Scully, C. Non-A, non-B hepatitis in dentistry. *Br. Dent. J.*, 1990;**168**:257–61.

[29] Samaranayake, L. P. Staff at risk from CMV. *The Dentist*, 1987;**4**:26–7.

[30] Smith, W.H.R. Intraoral and pulmonary tuberculosis following dental treatment. *Lancet*, 1988;**2**:824–44.

[31] Manton, S. L., Egglestone, S. I., Alexander, I., Scully, C. Oral presentation of secondary syphilis. *Br. Dent. J.*, 1986;**160**:237–8.

[32] Schuster, G. S. *Oral Microbiology and Infectious Diseases*. Baltimore/London, Williams and Wilkins, 1983.

[33] Thomas, L. E., Sydiskis, R. J., Devore, D. T., Krywolap, G. N. Survival of herpes simplex virus and other selected micro-organisms on patient charts: potential source of infection. *JAMA*, 1985;**111**:461–4.

[34] Manzella, J. R., McConville, J. H., Valenti, W., Megegus, M. A., Swierkosz, E. M., Arens, M. An outbreak of herpes simplex virus I gingivostomatitis in a dental hygiene practice. *JAMA*, 1984;**252**:2019–22.

[35] Rowe, N. H., Heine, C. S., Kowalski, C. J. Herpetic whitlow: an occupational disease in practising dentists. *J. Am. Dent. Assoc.*, 1982;**105**:471–3.

[36] Allen, A. L. and Organ, R. J. Occult blood under the fingernails: a mechanism for the spread of blood-borne infection. *J. Am. Dent. Assoc.*, 1982;**105**:449–55.

Further reading

More detailed information on HIV infection, AIDS, and oral manifestations of HIV infection is available in the following publications:

Farthing, C. F., Brown, S. E., Staughton, R. C. D. *A Colour Atlas of AIDS,* 2nd edn. London, Wolfe Medical Publications, 1988.
Barr, C. E. and Marder, M. Z. *AIDS, A Guide for Dental Practice.* Quintessence Int. Co. Inc., 1987.
Greenspan, D., Greenspan, J. S., Pinder, J. J. *et al. AIDS and the Dental Team,* Munsgaard, Copenhagen.

3. Objectives and Strategy

This chapter outlines the objectives, risks, and strategy involved in cross infection control.

General Objectives

The general aims of cross infection control are listed in **Table 3.1**.

Table 3.1   Objectives of Cross Infection Control.

- To protect the patient and members of the dental team from contracting infections during dental procedures.
- To reduce the numbers of pathogenic microorganisms in the dental environment, and therefore during dental procedures, to *the lowest possible level*.

- To implement a high standard of cross infection control when treating *every patient* (**universal precautions**), to prevent the transmission of infection.
- To simplify cross infection control, thus allowing the dental team to complete dental procedures with *minimal inconvenience*.

General Risks

To achieve these objectives the main risks must be identified (**3.1–3.7**).

1

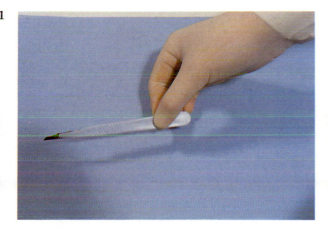

3.1   Risks from contaminated instruments.

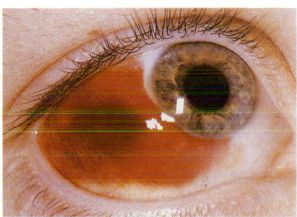

3.2   Risks from eye injury and subsequent infection. (Courtesy Dr M. V. Martin.)

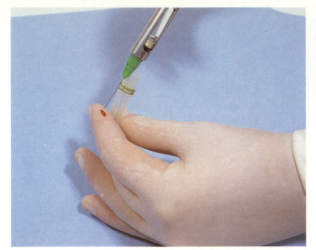

3.3 Risks from hand skin injury and infection.

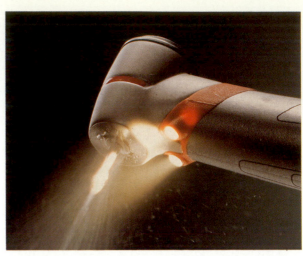

3.4 Risks from contaminated droplets and splatter. (Courtesy Siemens.)

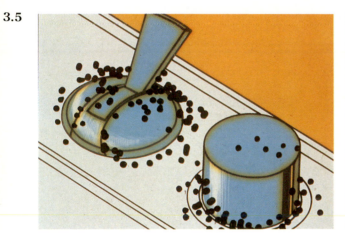

3.5 Risks from contaminated surfaces. (Courtesy Castellini.)

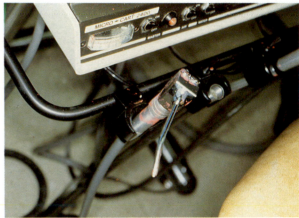

3.6 Risks from contaminated dental equipment. (Courtesy Drs J. Molinari and J. Young.)

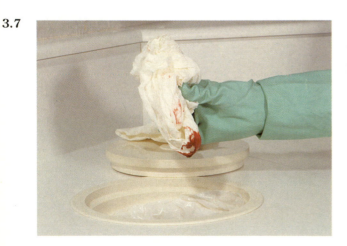

3.7 Risks from contaminated waste.

From a knowledge of such risks, a **strategy** must be formulated, to achieve the **objectives** of cross infection control. Such a strategy is detailed in **Table 3.2.**

Table 3.2   Strategy to achieve cross infection control.

- **All patients must be screened.**

- **Members of the dental team must stay healthy.**
  Consider:
  - Immunisation
  - Handwashing and handcare
  - Personal hygiene

- **Provide barriers for personal protection.**
  Consider:
  - Gloves
  - Masks
  - Eye protection
  - Clinical attire

- **Practise careful aseptic techniques,** limiting the spread of blood and saliva. Consider:
  - Handling of sharp instruments
  - Limiting surface contact:
    - The concept of unit dose, using surface disinfectants, drapes and covers, general surgery cleaning
  - Minimising aerosols and splatter by using:
    - Pre-operative mouthwashes
    - High-volume aspiration
    - The rubber dam
    - Ventilation and air filtration
  - Disposable items
  - Laundry of contaminated uniforms and linen
  - Handling of biopsy specimens and extracted teeth

- **Organise instruments carefully.** Consider:
  - Tray systems
  - Packaging instruments, sterilisation pouches

- **Sterilise** or disinfect all instruments and items used during dental procedures. Consider:
  - Holding solutions
    - Pre-sterilisation cleaning
    - Sterilisation
    - Testing sterilisation equipment
    - Aseptic storage
    - The sterilisation area
    - Instrument disinfection

- **Minimise possible contamination from dental equipment.** Consider:
  - The dental unit, chair and cabinetry
  - The dental unit water supply
  - Anti-retraction valves
  - Triple syringes
  - Ultrasonic scalers
  - Handpieces
  - The compressor

- **Dispose of contaminated waste safely.**
  Consider:
  - All clinical waste
  - Contaminated sharps
  - Liquid waste
  - The suction trap

- **Careful laboratory asepsis.**

- **Careful asepsis in radiology.**

- **Special care when undertaking endodontic procedures.**

- **Provide a written infection control programme,** staff training, periodic evaluation and updating of cross infection control procedures, and maintain careful records.

- **Understand national and local guidelines and regulations**

All the strategies listed in **Table 3.2** must be implemented when providing universal cross infection control.

The strategy outlined forms the basis of the practical guidelines described in this book.

Critical, Semi-Critical, and Non-Critical Items

Sterilisation is the destruction of *all* micro-organisms, whether vegetative or pathogenic, including highly resistant bacterial and mycotic spores.

Disinfection is the removal or inactivation of *some* micro-organisms, but not all.

Sanitisation refers to the use of chemicals and processes that maintain the microbial flora at a safe public-health level. Sanitisation has limited applicability in dentistry.

It is impossible to sterilise all instruments, items, surfaces etc. that become contaminated during dental procedures.

The choice of decontamination regimes may be based on how an item or instrument will be used. The Centers for Disease Control (CDC) has defined instruments as *critical* (**3.8**), *semi-critical* (**3.9**) and *non-critical* (**3.10**).

Critical instruments

3.8

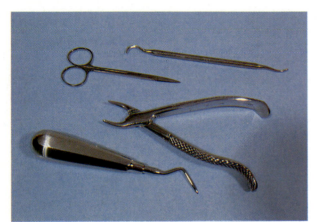

3.8 Critical instruments: scissors, forceps, elevator, and scaler.

If an instrument will be used to penetrate tissue or to touch bone (**3.8**) it *must* be sterilised.

Semi-critical instruments

3.9

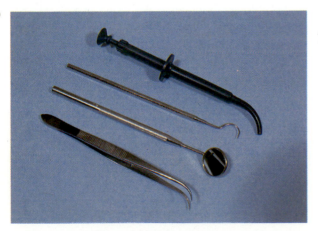

3.9 Semi-critical instruments: mirror, probe, amalgam carrier, and tweezers.

If an instrument will touch mucous membranes, but will not be used to penetrate tissue or to touch bone (**3.9**), it should be *sterilised* if at all possible or, if the instrument is susceptible to heat damage, it should be subjected to *high-level disinfection*.

Non-critical instruments

These are defined as equipment and surfaces which contact only intact skin (**3.10**), such as mixing slabs and spatulas. Work surfaces are decontaminated by using *intermediate-level disinfection*.

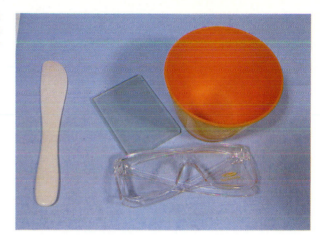

3.10

3.10 Non-critical instruments: spatula, mixing slab, and protective eyewear.

Summary

- Heat sterilise all critical instruments and semi-critical instruments which are not damaged by heat.
- Semi-critical instruments damaged by heat may be treated after use by high-level disinfection.
- Non-critical environmental surfaces are decontaminated using intermediate-level disinfection.

Categories of Tasks, Work Areas, and Personnel

The OSHA guidelines evaluate and classify tasks undertaken in a dental practice into one of three categories.

Category I: tasks that involve exposure to blood, body fluids, or tissues. All procedures or other job-related tasks that involve an inherent potential for contact of mucous membrane or skin with blood, body fluids, or tissues, or a potential for spills or splashes of these. Every employee engaged in category I tasks should be required to use appropriate protective measures.

Most, although not necessarily all, tasks performed by the dentist, oral hygienist, chairside assistant and laboratory technician would fall into this category.

Category II: tasks that involve no exposure to blood, body fluids or tissues, but personnel carrying out these tasks may be required to perform unplanned Category I tasks.

The normal work routine of these personnel involves no exposure to blood, body fluids or tissues, but the understanding that exposure or potential exposure may be required is a condition of employment. Every employee engaged in Category II tasks should have appropriate protective measures readily available.

Tasks performed by clerical or non-professional workers who may, as part of their duties, help to clean up the office, handle instruments or impression materials, or send out dental materials to laboratories, would be classified as Category II.

Category III: tasks that involve no exposure to blood, body fluids or tissues.

The normal work routine of these personnel involves no exposure to blood, body fluids or tissues. They are not called upon, as part of their employment, to perform or assist in emergency medical care or first aid, or to be potentially exposed in some other way.

A front-office receptionist, book-keeper, or insurance clerk who does not handle dental instruments or materials would be a Category III worker.

Note: These classifications are not rigid and there may be crossover, depending upon the job performed.

4. Patient Screening

It is essential to screen *all* patients. This includes a full medical history, a social history, and a soft-tissue examination.

Screening identifies some *unknown carriers* of infectious disease and achieves the following:

- *Early* diagnosis of disease.
- *Early* treatment of previously undiagnosed conditions.
- *Early* availability of counselling by experienced persons.
- Modification of infection control if the patient is medically compromised, e.g. availability of sterile water for dental procedures.

But note: *identification* of a carrier of an infectious disease *does not* imply that *special infection control* precautions should be taken *only* when a patient is medically compromised.

Medical History

A thorough medical history should be taken from each new patient and *updated* at subsequent appointments. The patient should sign and date the medical-history sheet.

The patient history is unreliable in identifying the incidence of past infections. It has been shown that four out of five individuals who have had hepatitis B were not completely diagnosed and therefore would not report this on their medical history.[1]

Some carriers of an infectious disease may not disclose this fact, for fear of being refused treatment.

General inclusions

Include: past history of illness; surgery; hospital care; injections received, especially in third world countries; current medications; allergies; adverse drug reactions; and transfusions.

Always use a medical-history sheet recommended by your Dental Association, e.g. ADA, BDA, etc.

Specific additional questions

Ask about a history of the infectious diseases listed in **Table 4.1**. This list may be incorporated into the medical questionnaire.

Certain characteristics may suggest HIV infection,[2] especially if occurring simultaneously. These are listed in **Table 4.2**. Include this list in the medical questionnaire.

Table 4.1   Diseases of concern.

AIDS
Hepatitis B
Hepatitis C
Tuberculosis
Herpes
Measles
Infectious neurological and respiratory diseases
Infectious mononucleosis (glandular fever)
Gonorrhoea
Syphilis

Table 4.2   Characteristics suggesting HIV infection.

Fever of unknown origin
Night sweats
Weight loss (unexplained)
Recurrent infections
Soft-tissue lesions
Unexplained lymphadenopathy
Long-standing chronic diarrhoea

Patients infected with HIV may suffer medium to severe **immunosuppression** and increased susceptibility to a variety of infectious diseases. There are *other* causes of immunosuppression (**Table 4.3**) which should be listed in a medical questionnaire and *eliminated* before HIV infection is suspected.

Table 4.3   Causes of immunosuppression.

Cause	Examples
Physiological	Neonates, old age
Drug-induced	Cytotoxic drugs, antimetabolic agents
Autoimmune disease	Diabetes mellitus, rheumatoid arthritis
Malignant disease	Leukaemia, Hodgkin's disease
Radiotherapy	

From: *Infection Control in the Dental Environment.* (With permission from Dr M. V. Martin.)

Social History

The second section of the questionnaire should include questions relevant to the patient's lifestyle. Allow the patient to study the list in **Tables 4.4** and **4.5** and encourage further discussion if necessary.

Areas having a high incidence of HIV (**4.1**) and hepatitis B (**4.2**) are illustrated. Persons who have regularly visited or have been resident in these areas may be included in high-risk groups for HBV or HIV infection.

Table 4.4   Groups at high risk for HIV infection.

Homosexual and bisexual males
Intravenous drug abusers
Transfusion recipients
Infants born to infected mothers
Heterosexual contacts of infected individuals

Table 4.5   Groups at high risk for hepatitis B infection.

Intravenous drug abusers
Homosexual and bisexual males
Heterosexually active persons with multiple sexual contacts
Persons living and working in institutions
Patients who have spent their lives in highly endemic areas
Patients with acute or chronic liver disease
Recipients of unscreened blood
Healthcare personnel
Oncology and dialysis patients
Household members and sexual contacts of HBV carriers
Infants born to HBV-positive mothers
International travellers to areas with a HBV epidemic

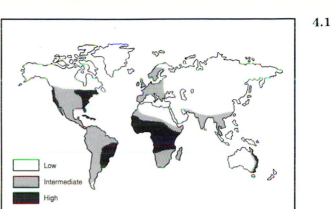

4.1 Areas with a high incidence of HIV. (Courtesy Prof. C. Scully and the *British Dental Journal*.)

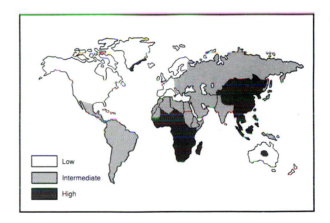

4.2 Areas with a high incidence of hepatitis B. (Courtesy Prof. C. Scully and the *British Dental Journal*.)

Soft-Tissue Examination

A thorough examination of the soft tissues may reveal oral manifestations of HIV infection, which may identify a previously unknown carrier of the disease. Further information is included in Chapter 2 (p. 17).

Points to remember

- Use a printed medical- and social-history questionnaire and explain the reasons for requesting the relevant information.
- Assure patients that they will *not* be denied treatment if they are identified as a carrier of an infectious disease.
- Allow the patient sufficient time to complete the questionnaire *in private*.
- Discuss the patient's misgivings or reservations, after the questionnaire is completed — *in private*.

- Treat all information as *confidential*. Emphasise that members of staff *never* discuss such confidential information within the hearing of other patients, over the telephone, or outside the practice. Records should be filed in locked cabinets, and only certain staff members should have access to such records.
- The dentist should consult with the patient's physician (with the patient's written permission), following disclosure of information which may suggest further investigation, medical treatment or counselling.

References

[1]Cottone, J. A. Hepatitis B virus infection and the dental profession. *J. Am. Dent. Assoc.*, 1985; **110**:617–21.
[2]Greenspan, D., Greenspan, J. S., Pindborg, J. J., Schiodt, M. *Aids and the Dental Team,* Copenhagen; Munksgaard, 1986.

5. Staying Healthy

Immunisation

Immunisation reduces the risk to dental healthcare workers of becoming infected and may also protect their patients and family. The following should be vaccinated:

Dentists
Hygienists
Dental surgery assistants
Laboratory technicians
Engineers who repair dental equipment.

Vaccines available are listed in **Table 5.1**.

All groups at risk should complete a questionnaire such as that illustrated in **Table 5.2**. Dentists should issue written advice to all clinical staff recommending immunisation against the infectious diseases listed.

Table 5.1 Vaccines available to dental healthcare workers.

Hepatitis B
Influenza
Mumps
Measles
Tetanus
Rubella (German measles)
Poliomyelitis
Whooping cough
Tuberculosis

Table 5.2 Questionnaire to be completed by all dental healthcare workers.

Name: Position:

Disease	Have you had the disease?	Are you immunised?	Do you require immunisation?
Hepatitis B			
Influenza			
Mumps			
Measles			
Polio			
Tetanus			
Rubella			
Whooping cough			
Tuberculosis			

If you have had these diseases or have been immunised against them you should be **immune**. *If you are not immune you may acquire these infections from an infected patient. Pregnancy and certain health conditions may mean that these recommendations should be modified. IF IN DOUBT, PLEASE CONSULT YOUR PHYSICIAN.*

Tetanus

Dental healthcare workers should be immunised against tetanus and they should maintain that protection with boosters every **5 years**.

Rubella

Female staff of childbearing age who are not immune, should receive the rubella vaccine, since contracting German measles during pregnancy results in a high incidence of foetal abnormalities, including deafness and mental retardation. Vaccination against rubella should be avoided if already pregnant.

Influenza

Immunisation against influenza may:

- Help avoid loss of work time and inconvenience.
- Avoid the healthcare worker giving patients influenza.

Immunity produced by this vaccine *is not permanent*. A person should be immunised each autumn with the updated vaccine formulated against the current biotypes of the virus.

Poliomyelitis

An oral vaccine is available which gives protection for 5 years.

Tuberculosis

A subdermal vaccine is available. The recipient should be re-tested every 5 years.

Hepatitis B

Dental healthcare workers are at high risk of acquiring hepatitis B through contact with patients. A survey conducted between 1983 and 1985[1], found that 14% of dentists tested for HBV serum markers showed evidence of natural immunity. The chronic carrier rate was 0.94%, which was consistent with earlier findings.

In 1988, the percentage of dentists with natural immunity had dropped to 8.58%. The increase in the number of dentists receiving hepatitis B vaccine accounted for this decrease.[2]

The American Dental Association (ADA) Council on Dental Therapeutics, Immunisation Practices Advisory Committee (IPAC), Centers for Disease Control (CDC), British Dental Association (BDA), and the majority of dental associations throughout the world *strongly* recommend that dental healthcare workers are vaccinated against hepatitis B.

Immunisation against hepatitis B is *essential* for *all* dental healthcare workers.

Two types of vaccines are available:

- Recombivax HB: the first recombinant-DNA vaccine.
- Engerix B: the latest recombinant-DNA vaccine.

OSHA instruction—USA

The current Occupational Safety and Health Administration (OSHA) instruction states:

'The facilities for infection control policy regarding hepatitis B vaccinations shall address all circumstances warranting such vaccinations and shall identify employees at substantial risk of directly contacting body fluids. All such employees shall be offered hepatitis B vaccinations *free of charge* in amounts and at times prescribed by standard medical practice.'

That is, employers are required to pay for HBV vaccination and must inform employees of the availability of the vaccine, the benefits of vaccination, and where the vaccine can be obtained.

HBV vaccination policy
Employers should provide a written statement of their policy with regard to hepatitis B vaccination. If an employee elects *not* to receive HBV vaccination, after reading such a statement and *understanding* the benefits of vaccination, then the employee should complete an **informed refusal form**.

New members of staff
At present, OSHA states that it is permissible for a new trainee employee to conduct patient care during the 2–6 month period it takes to complete the necessary series of vaccine injections.

Note: It may be preferable for a new member of staff to receive an accelerated dose of vaccine, and not to assist in clinical procedures for the first 2 months.

Vaccination procedure

Pre-testing

The vaccine need not be given to individuals known to be hepatitis B surface *antigen* or *antibody* positive, i.e. with an anti-HB level over 100 iu/l. However, pretesting may not be necessary or cost effective, as only 6.7% of vaccine recipients in dentistry are already immune.[3]

Immunisation

The vaccine is highly efficacious, giving up to 95% sero-conversion. The immunisation regimen is:

First dose—elected date.
Second dose—1 month later.
Third dose—6 months after the first dose.

For more rapid immunisation using the **recombinant** vaccine, the *third* dose may be given 2 months after the initial dose, with a booster at 12 months. This is very useful for new members of staff.

In adults, the injection is given intramuscularly in the **deltoid region**, because when given in the gluteds sero-conversion does not occur in some cases.

Post-vaccination screening

Screening for antibody response is carried out 2–4 months after the last injection of vaccine (never later than 6 months after the last injection). Non-responders should be given three more doses of vaccine. Only 55% of non-responders sero-convert.[4] Non-responders who are healthcare workers should consult their physician with a view to obtaining specialist advice.

Booster doses

The duration of immunity is not precisely known, but is in the order of 3–5 years. A booster dose should be given after this period, since after 5 years only 75% of individuals have adequate antibody levels.[5,6]

Individuals who are at risk may wish to determine their antibody level periodically. If this level falls below 100 iu/l, they should consider the need for a booster dose.[7]

In some countries (e.g. Germany), the time interval between initial immunisation and the follow-up test for the level of antibodies, is determined by the level of serum antibodies at the initial post-vaccination test. The following recommendations have been made:

- If anti-HBs levels are below 100 iu/l at the initial post-vaccination test—re-vaccinate within 6 months.
- If anti-HBs levels are 101–1000 iu/l—test after 2–4 years.
- If anti-HBs levels are above 1000 iu/l—test after 4–6 years.

Individuals who lose a detectable antibody titre may have a secondary *anamnestic* response which protects against clinical infection.[3] Therefore it is possible that the immediate boosting of titres falling below 100 iu/l may not be essential.

Immunisation during pregnancy

Hepatitis B infection during pregnancy may result in severe disease of the mother and chronic infection of the newborn. CDC states:

'Although there is no risk to the foetus if the vaccine is given, immunisation during pregnancy is not routinely recommended, and therefore always consult the dental healthcare worker's physician.'

Hand Care

Hand skin

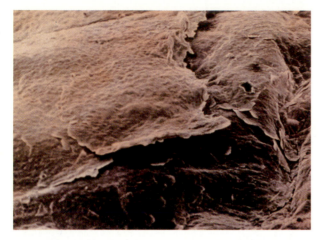

5.1 Skin magnified to show skin squamae (×250). (Courtesy ICI.)

5.2 Scanning electron micrograph of skin showing bacteria lying on individual squamae (×4000). (Courtesy ICI.)

The surface of hand skin, the stratum corneum, is made up of minute plates—the squamae, which are flat sheets of dead epithelial cells (keratin) (**5.1**). These are shed continuously and are replaced through cell division in lower layers of the skin.

The stratum corneum provides the main barrier-effect of the skin and, if damaged, provides a portal of entry for pathogenic micro-organisms. The surface of the skin is bathed by two 'conditioning' fluids:

- **Perspiration** from the sweat glands—mainly water.
- **Sebum**—an oily fluid produced by sebaceous glands.

The presence of perspiration and sebum keeps the stratum corneum in good condition. The combination of the two fluids maintains a constant level of acidity (pH 5.5–6.5) on the skin surface and under these conditions the keratin is a strong, smooth, impervious material. At a higher pH (8 or 9), keratin becomes weak, and the surface becomes rough and relatively porous.[8]

Hand skin contains two types of microflora. **Resident** micro-organisms (**5.2**) are those that survive and multiply on the skin and can be repeatedly cultured. **Transient** micro-organisms are recent contaminants, that remain on the skin for limited periods. Most of the resident micro-organisms are found on the top layers of the skin; however, some are found in deeper layers. Many resident micro-organisms are not highly infectious, but may be implicated in skin infections and opportunistic infections. Some can cause infections in patients when invasive procedures, such as surgery, allow them to enter oral mucous membrane or bone, or when a patient is medically compromised.

Skin cleaning

Hand washing removes blood, debris, and contaminating micro-organisms, but may damage the skin.

Correct hand washing should maintain the pH balance of the skin, and maintain the keratin condition and the production of perspiration and sebum.

Many soaps have a pH of at least 9. After multiple washes, such alkalinity alters the surface pH, resulting in skin roughness and redness. It is, therefore, important to choose a handwash based on a detergent with a pH similar to that of the skin.

Many antibacterial handwashes contain chlorhexidine 4% or other antiseptics. Multiple hand washing with these products may remove sebum and result in dry, sore, skin. Reconditioning creams help to overcome such a problem.

Skin damage

If gloves are not worn, hands become contaminated with blood during dental procedures. Remnants of blood have been found under the nails of the thumbs and index fingers of 80% of dentists, and 40% had blood on their hands after the weekend.[9]

Although the majority of dentists now wear operating gloves, their hands may still contact blood if gloves are faulty or become damaged during the dental procedure. Intact hand skin prevents possible invasion by pathogenic micro-organisms, following hand contact with blood. However, damaged hand skin allows entry of pathogenic micro-organisms, and presents a risk of infection to the dental healthcare worker. In addition, damaged hand skin may encourage the proliferation of pathogenic micro-organisms, which could be hazardous if transmitted to immuno-compromised patients. Dentists should have a basic knowledge of causes of hand skin damage and conditions affecting hand skin.

Physical damage

The usual causes are:
- Cuts and grazes during activities outside work, e.g. DIY, sport, gardening, etc. Care should be taken to protect the hands during these activities, e.g. wear heavy protective gloves if possible.
- Burns from the Bunsen burner.

Dermatitis

There are three distinct types of dermatitis: irritant contact dermatitis (ICD), allergic contact dermatitis (ACD), and contact urticaria (CU).

Irritant contact dermatitis

5.3

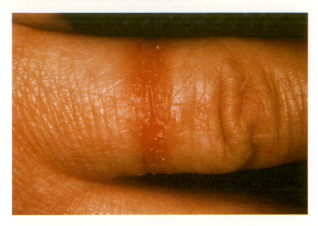

5.3 Irritant contact dermatitis: red, scaly, fissured skin under a ring. (Courtesy Dr E. A. Field and the *British Dental Journal*.)

5.4

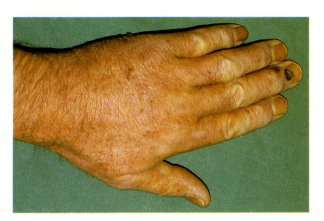

5.4 Chronic contact dermatitis: there is a marked scaling, thickening, and fissuring of the skin. (Courtesy Dr W. J. Cunliffe.)

This involves direct damage to the stratum corneum by toxic chemicals, such as soaps, detergents, and acids and alkalis.

There are several exacerbating factors including:

- Sweating.
- Occlusion (e.g. by gloves).
- High humidity.
- Heat.
- Low humidity.
- Cold.

ICD is particularly associated with wet work. Inadequate rinsing and drying of the hands allows residues of soap or detergent to remain under rings or between the fingers, where they initiate irritation. The wearing of gloves may exacerbate this as there may be a tendency to excessive sweating (hyperhidrosis).

Acute ICD is caused by contact with a single strong irritant, which produces burning or blistering at the contact site.

Chronic ICD is caused by repeated contact with weaker chemicals over a period of time.

Initially, ICD appears as 'chapping', i.e. itchy, dry, fissured skin under a ring, or on the finger webs or dorsa of the hands (**5.3**). Greater degrees of irritation will result in redness, thickening, and fissuring of the skin (**5.4**).

Prevention and Management of ICD

- Hands should be carefully rinsed and dried after washing. Avoid hot water for washing.
- Emollients, e.g. emulsifying ointment or aqueous cream, should be used as soap substitutes, at home and at work.
- Moisturising cream, such as Neutrogena Norwegian formula handcream, Vaseline Dermacare, or E45, should be applied after hand washing.
- Gloves should be removed frequently, to overcome sweating.

- Hyperhidrosis of the palms may respond to aluminium chloride hexahydrate 20% in ethanol (Anhydrol Forte Drichlor). This should be applied from a roll bottle at night, allowed to dry, and washed off in the morning. However, it may irritate broken skin.
- Silk glove liners (Sensi Touch) are available. These absorb sweat and reduce friction.
- Irritant chemicals should be handled while wearing protective heavy rubber gloves.

Allergic contact dermatitis (ACD)

This is a true allergy, manifesting as dermatitis at the site of contact, possibly later becoming widespread. Once acquired, the allergy tends to persist indefinitely. The diagnosis is confirmed by patch testing (**5.5**).

Common sensitisers found in dentistry include:

- Acrylate and methacrylate monomers.
- Catalysts in dental impression materials.
- Essential oils (e.g. cinnamon oil, eugenol, clove oil).
- Rubber additives.
- Antiseptic detergents (e.g. those containing benzalkonium chloride).
- Formaldehyde.
- Mercury.
- Nickel.

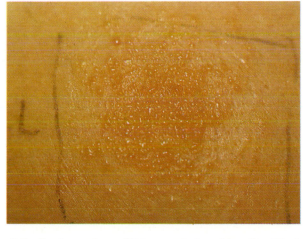

5.5 Patch testing. (With permission from Dr W. J. Cunliffe.)

Allergy and Latex Gloves

Rubber is a contact allergen that causes skin sensitisation. When latex is vulcanised, **accelerators**, which speed up the process of vulcanisation, and **antioxidants**, which prolong the life of the rubber, are used.

Accelerators, e.g. thiurams, dithiocarbamates, and guanidines, are the usual cause of ACD from wearing latex gloves. However, this condition is rare.

Clinical features of ACD

These include a *sharply delineated* band of eczema on the forearm, which corresponds to the upper border of the glove; or a definite patchy eczema of the fingers (**5.6**).

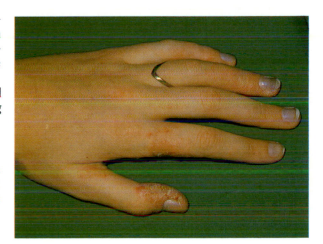

5.6 Allergic contact dermatitis. (With permission from Dr W.J. Cunliffe.)

Management of ACD

Remove contact with the allergen involved. In the case of allergy to latex gloves:

- Switch to hypoallergenic gloves, containing a low residue of dithiocarbamate and *no thiurams*.
- If the eczema persists, use PVC vinyl gloves, or latex rubber gloves which are manufactured by a special process which avoids all vulcanising materials (e.g. Puritee hypoallergenic latex gloves) or artificial rubber gloves made of styrene-butadiene monomer (e.g. Elastyren).

Contact urticaria

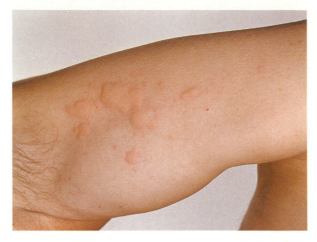

5.7 Urticarial wheals on the skin. (With permission from Dr W. J. Cunliffe.)

This is a wheal and flare reaction to contact of the skin with a substance which stimulates the release of histamine. CU is becoming increasingly common, due to a protein in natural latex.

Symptoms occur either within minutes of, or a few hours after, wearing rubber gloves. Occasionally, itching of the hands and wrists may be the only reaction, however, often there may be swelling or wheals on the skin which was contacting the gloves. This resolves within a short time of glove removal (**5.7**).

It is essential to recognise this condition at an early stage to avoid more serious reactions such as urticaria, tachycardia, breathlessness, and anaphylactic shock. Early testing for CU is strongly advised, and those who are affected by rubber-induced CU, no matter how mild, should avoid all contact with rubber products.

Paronychia

Paronychia is a superinfection by pathogens of damaged macerated skin around the nail.

Acute Paronychia

This is usually a staphyloccoccal infection of the nail fold. Most cases result from local trauma. The nail fold becomes swollen and painful, and pus may be present.

Cleaning and washing may resolve the condition, otherwise systemic antibiotics e.g. flucloxacillin may be necessary. Recalcitrant lesions may require incision and drainage.

Chronic Paronychia

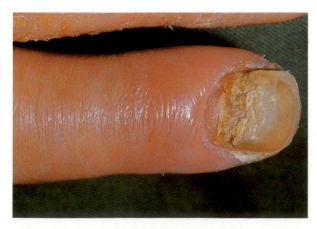

Infection of the nail fold with *Candida* (**5.8**). This condition may occur when the hands are continually exposed to water, or when latex gloves are worn for long periods.

Hands should be kept dry. Regular use of topical Nystatin or an imidazole cream or lotion (e.g. econazole, clotrimazole or miconazole) is recommended. A bacterial superinfection may have to be treated. This may be difficult if the skin is continually covered by impervious materials, e.g. through glove wearing.

5.8 Chronic paronychia: there is swelling of the nail fold, loss of the cuticle, and distortion of the nail plate. (With permission from Dr W. J. Cunliffe.)

Psoriasis

Psoriatic lesions are not due to infection. The hands, when involved, become red, with thickening of the keratin layer, scaling, and sometimes pustulation (**5.9**). When the condition is severe, the skin may be sore and fissured, and the nails pitted, discoloured, and thickened (**5.10**). The skin may be affected by irritants and wet work.

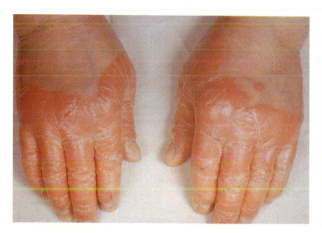

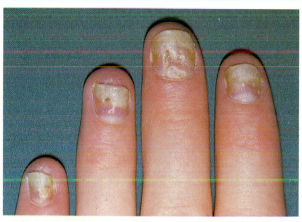

5.9   Psoriasis of the hands. (Courtesy Dr W. J. Cunliffe.)

5.10   Nail psoriasis: the nail plate is virtually destroyed. (Courtesy Dr W. J. Cunliffe.)

Summary and recommendations

It is important that skin conditions are identified at an early stage, and immediate investigation by a dermatologist is strongly recommended.

Hand skin damage may be avoided if sensible precautions are taken by dental healthcare workers. Recommendations are summarised in **Table 5.3**.

Table 5.3   Precautions necessary to avoid hand skin damage

- Change to a different product if any disinfectants, hand washing solutions, or soaps cause skin irritation.
- Remove all rings and jewellery before washing, as irritants may accumulate under these.
- Rinse hands with *cool* water. Hot water opens the skin pores. Cool water prevents debris from penetrating the skin pores, and minimises the shedding of resident micro-organisms from the sub-surface layers of the skin.
- Dry hands thoroughly after washing.
- Change protective gloves regularly to avoid a build up of sweat.
- Use a good quality moisturising cream regularly after each clinical session.
- Minimise skin contact with potentially sensitising chemicals or medicaments. Some may penetrate rubber, e.g. acrylic monomers and nickel.
- Wear heavy work gloves when undertaking work outside the surgery which is likely to damage the hands.
- Keep fingernails short and well manicured, and avoid wearing nail varnish or false fingernails at work.
- Protect cuts or abrasions on the hands or forearms, with a waterproof dressing, before undertaking dental procedures.
- Dental personnel who have widespread exudative or weeping dermatitis, which cannot be protected, should refrain from all direct patient care, and from handling contaminated equipment.

Hand Washing

Hand washing removes debris, blood, and potentially pathogenic transient micro-organisms from the hands, and achieves two general objectives:

- To destroy pathogenic micro-organisms which collect on the hands while providing dental treat- ment, thus avoiding transmission to other patients.
- To prevent blood which contains pathogenic micro-organisms from accumulating on damaged hand skin and transmitting infection to the dental healthcare worker.

General principles

Mechanical removal of debris and of transient micro-organisms

Hand washing procedure is *very* important and may be more important than the type of soap used. Each part of the hand washing process is necessary to remove micro-organisms.

- Rubbing removes micro-organisms from the skin.
- Lathering holds them suspended away from the skin's surface.
- Rinsing washes them off the hands.

Disinfection

The disinfectant action of hand washing will destroy *in situ* micro-organisms on the surface of the hands.

In the UK, USA, and Scandinavia, it is accepted that both removal and disinfection are part of a complete hand wash.

Hand washing and gloves

Hand washing before gloving is intended to remove transient micro-organisms, and to suppress residual micro-flora while wearing the gloves. This provides protection for the patient and the user, if gloves are torn, and prevents hand irritation caused by excessive growth of residual micro-flora. Hand washing after glove removal is intended to remove micro-organisms, which may have penetrated the gloves through microscopic defects or tears, and to reduce any residual micro-flora build up that may have occurred.

Handscrubs and handwashes

Surgical handscrubs

These are preparations that significantly reduce the number of micro-organisms present on intact skin. A surgical handscrub should:

- Act fast
- Not irritate the skin after repeated use
- Have a broad range of bactericidal and residual activity.

Many products are categorised as both a surgical handscrub and a healthcare personnel handwash; the activity being determined by the length of time the handwash is used. For example, to use 4% chlorhexidine gluconate with 4% isopropyl alcohol as:

- A surgical handscrub: 2 consecutive 3-minute scrubs.
- A healthcare personnel handwash: 2 × 15-second hand washes.

Products currently accepted by the Council on Dental Therapeutics (CDT) are described in the ADA publication, *Clinical Products in Dentistry: a Desktop Reference.*

Healthcare personnel handwashes

These handwashes are non-irritating, anti-microbial preparations designed for frequent use. Labelling of the product, e.g. 'reduces skin flora', 'reduces cross infection risks', 'fast acting', and 'broad spectrum', should be supported by data from handwashing studies.

Healthcare personnel handwashes have bacteriostatic or germicidal ingredients which have been shown to be active against residual skin microflora or transient micro-organisms. Suppression of bacterial counts makes these cleaners especially suited for washing before gloving.

Other types of hand cleansers

General soaps may cause excessive dryness or defatting of the hands and may be extremely irritating for extensive daily use in dentistry and other healthcare settings. Hand cleaners labelled 'mild', 'gentle', 'lotion', and 'non-irritating' are formulated to be non-irritating, to minimise fat removal from the hands or,

to re-lubricate the skin. They can also reduce the breakdown of skin components and preserve the skin pH when there is extensive repeated use. These cleansers do not necessarily contain active anti-bacterials unless so labelled.

Antiseptics used in hand washing

Chlorhexidine

This is 2–4% chlorhexidine gluconate with 4% isopropyl alcohol in a detergent solution with a pH of 5.0 to 6.5. Recent studies indicate that chlorhexidine handwash is more effective than povidone iodine or parachlorometexylenol (PCMX).[10,11]

Povidone iodine

These products contain 7.5% to 10% povidone iodine, providing 0.75% to 1.00% available iodine. Products containing emollients are available, for repeated use as healthcare personnel handwashes. For use as a surgical handscrub, use two consecutive scrubs of 3-minute duration.

Phenolic compounds

Hexachlorophene can be absorbed into the blood stream through intact skin, although it is more readily absorbed through abraded skin. It may be toxic if the blood concentration rises with repeated exposure.

Parachlorometexylenol (PCMX) is bactericidal and fungicidal at 2% concentration. It does not appear to be toxic.

Alcohols

Ethyl alcohol and isopropyl alcohol are widely used as topical skin antiseptics, and have a potent bactericidal effect, especially at 70% concentration.

Finger-tip cultures taken from the hands, before and after washing, are illustrated (**5.11–5.16**).

1

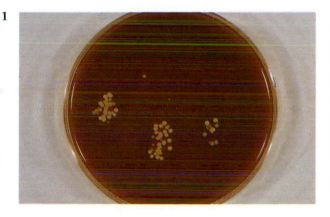

5.12

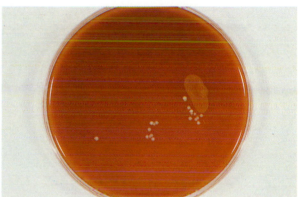

5.11, 5.12   Finger-tip cultures taken from the left and right hands before washing. (Courtesy Dr M. V. Martin.)

5.13

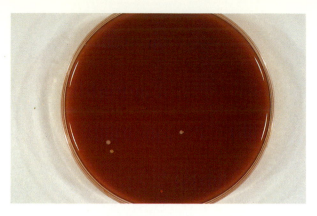 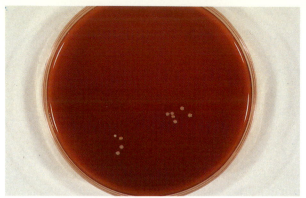

5.13, 5.14 Finger-tip cultures taken from the left and right hands after washing with chlorhexidine 4% (Hibiscrub). (Courtesy Dr M. V. Martin.)

5.15

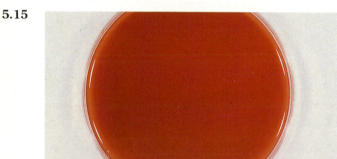 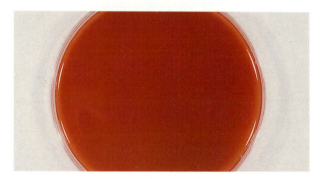

5.15, 5.16 Finger-tip cultures taken from the left and right hands after using an alcohol-based hand rub (Hibisol). (Courtesy Dr M. V. Martin.)

Note: Repeated use of the above bactericidal handwashes may cause skin irritation and subsequent damage. If this occurs, a different product should be used until a suitable non-irritant handwash is found.

Hand Washing Procedures

Full hand washing

To be carried out *before* and *after* each clinical session.

5.17

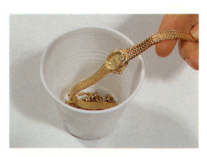 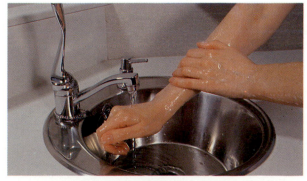

5.17 Remove jewellery and place item(s) in a safe container.

5.18 Preliminary hand and lower arm wash: Rinse the forearms and hands using cool water, and wash the hands and lower arms with a disinfectant handscrub for 15 seconds, rinse this off with cool water.

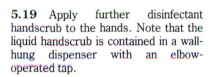

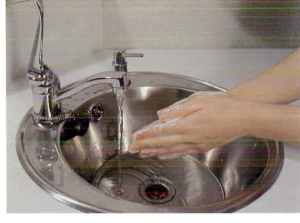

5.19 Apply further disinfectant handscrub to the hands. Note that the liquid handscrub is contained in a wall-hung dispenser with an elbow-operated tap.

5.20 Wash the palms of the hands.

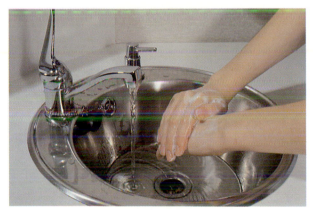

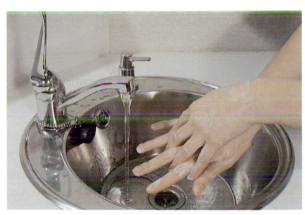

5.21 Wash the backs of the hands.

5.22 Wash the finger webs.

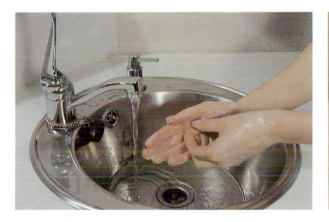

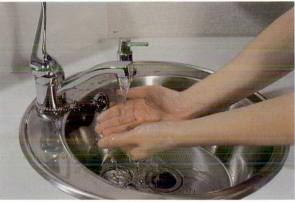

5.23 Wash the tips of the fingers and thumbs, especially around the nail area.

5.24 Rinse the hands thoroughly with cool water.

The full hand wash (**5.19–5.24**), which should last at least 15 seconds, is *repeated*.

5.25

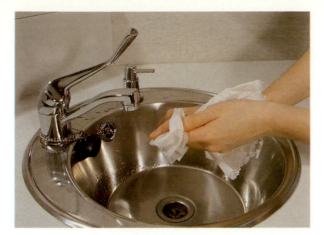

5.25 The hands and forearms are *thoroughly* dried with soft, good-quality, disposable paper towels.

5.26

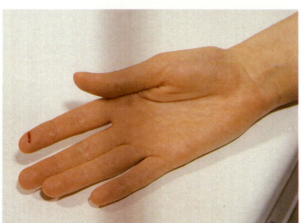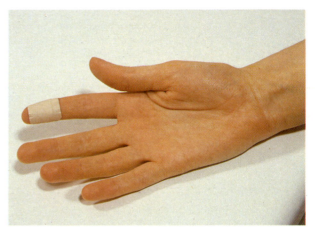

5.26, 5.27 Any hand cuts or abrasions are covered with a waterproof dressing.

5.28

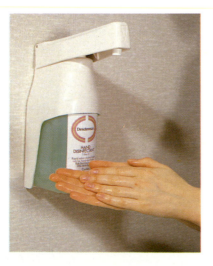

5.28 An alcohol-based disinfectant hand rub is then applied to the hands in the same manner as the liquid hand-scrub. This evaporates quickly, and when the hands are dry a pair of operating gloves is put on.

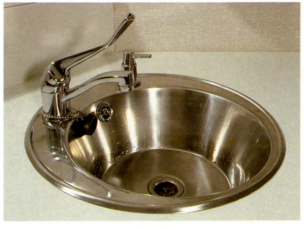

5.29 Elbow taps should be used.

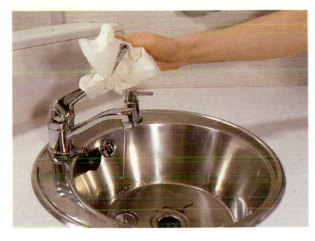

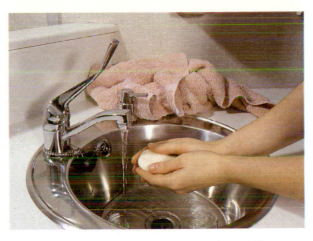

5.30 If a hand-operated faucet is used, do not touch the handle with bare skin. Use a clean paper towel to avoid contaminating the handle or your hands.

5.31 Do not use linen towels or bars of soap. These are inefficient and unhygienic.[8]

The surgical handscrub

Use the same technique as described for **full hand washing**, but the two separate washes should be carried out for the time specified in the surgical handscrub instructions (usually two 3-minute washes). Hands and forearms may be scrubbed using a *sterile* or *disposable* handbrush. Avoid over-vigourous scrubbing, especially around the fingernails and nailbeds, as skin damage may result. Dry the hands using sterile towels.

Between patients, or after changing damaged or worn-out gloves

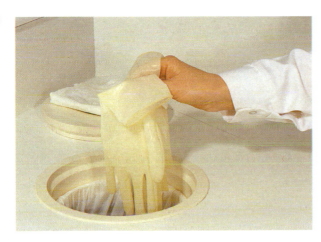

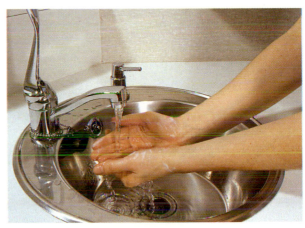

5.32 Discard the gloves used during the previous dental procedure.

5.33 Rinse the hands thoroughly with cool water, **and also the forearms if a short-sleeved coat is worn.**

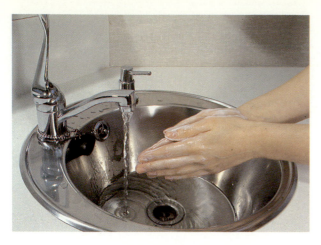

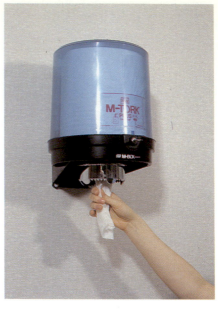

5.34 Wash the hands and forearms thoroughly for 15 seconds using a bactericidal liquid soap. If repeated use of healthcare personnel handwashes causes hand skin irritation, change to a mild hand cleanser. This wash removes sweat, glove chalk and micro-organisms from the forearms and hands. Then, rinse the hands and forearms thoroughly with cool water.

5.35 Dry the hands and forearms with good-quality, soft, disposable paper towels. Note that the type of dispenser illustrated facilitates towel removal without touching the dispenser.

5.36

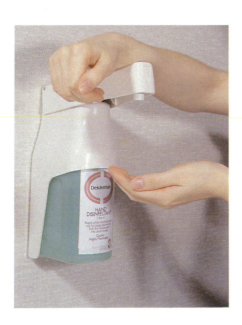

5.36 Apply an alcohol-based hand rub to the hands. If repeated, prolonged use of an alcohol-based hand rub causes hand skin irritation, try another product. Put on a new pair of operating gloves.

Recommended hand washing products (USA)

In 1987, Clinical Research Associates (CRA)[12] recommended the following products:

Steri stat	4% chlorhexidine	Liquid
Hibiclens/Hibiscrub	4% chlorhexidine	Liquid
Lurodine	0.75% available iodine	Liquid
Luroscrub	4% chlorhexidine	Liquid
Bactoshield II	2% chlorhexidine	Liquid

Other products now recommended are CHG (Dexide), Excelle, and Novoclens.

The recommended products have rapid microbial activity with residual and cumulative activity. The same study did not recommend handwashes containing 5% PCMX (Derm Aseptic) and 1% Tridosan (Ultraclean).

Alcare (54% ethanol) and TLC produce rapid antimicrobial activity alone and are recommended.

Hand creams

Kerodex 71 or Foam care are recommended.

Personal Hygiene

The following guidelines apply to all clinical dental healthcare workers who may come into contact with blood or body fluids:

- Hair should be short or kept away from the face.
- Facial hair should be covered with a face mask or shield.
- Jewellery should not be worn on the hands or arms during clinical sessions.
- Nails must be kept clean and short.

References

[1] Siew, C., Gruninger, S.E., Mitchell, E.W., Burrell, K.H. Survey of hepatitis B exposure and vaccination in volunteer dentists. *J. Am. Dent. Assoc.*, 1987; **114**: 457–9.

[2] Siew, C., Gruninger, S.E., Mitchell, E.W., Burrell, K.H. Risk of HIV and hepatitis B infection among dental professionals (abstract). *J. Dent. Res.*, 1989; **68**: 45–6.

[3] Cottone, J. Recent developments in hepatitis; new virus vaccine and dosage. Recommendations. *J. Am. Dent. Assoc.*, 1990; **120**: 501–8.

[4] Just, M., Berger, R., Andre, F., Sarary, A. Boosting against hepatitis B, must it be done when titres disappear. *In* Zuckerman, A.J. (ed.) *International symposium on viral hepatitis and liver disease,* Abstract **85A**; p.266, Turnhaut, Belgium: Organon Teckinka, 1987.

[5] Jacobsen, I.M. and Dines, L. Viral hepatitis vaccines. *Ann. Rev. Med.*, 1985; **37**: 241–61.

[6] Scully, C. Hepatitis B immunisation of dental students in 14 UK dental schools. *Br. Dent. J.*, 1989; **166**: 360.

[7] Scully, C., Cawson, R.A., Griffiths, M.J. *Occupational Hazards in Dentistry.* London. British Dental Journal, 1990.

[8] Field, E.A., Martin, M.V. Handwashing soap or disinfectant? *Br. Dent. J.*, 1986; **160**: 278–80.

[9] Allen, A.L. and Organ, R.J. Occult blood under the fingernails, a mechanism for the spread of blood-borne infections. *J. Am. Dent. Assoc.*, 1982; **105**: 455–9.

[10] Higbee, K., Robinson, R., Carter, M., Robinson, D., Christenson, R. Handwash study 87 (Unpublished data).

[11] Robinson, D., Robinson, R., Christenson, R. Comparison of four antimicrobial agents in handwashes. *J. Dent. Res.*, (Abstract), 1987; **66**: 335.

[12] Clinical Research Associates. Volume 2, Issue 5, May 1987.

6. Personal Protection

Personal Protective Barriers

Special protective coverings act as a barrier, protecting the dental healthcare worker from contact with blood, and saliva contaminated with blood.

Barriers considered *essential* when performing all dental procedures are: gloves, masks, protective eyewear, and protective uniforms.

Gloves

The main types of glove used in dentistry are:

- Latex gloves: non-sterile and sterile
- Vinyl gloves: non-sterile and sterile
- General-purpose utility gloves
- Surgeon's sterile gloves.

Latex gloves

The reasons for wearing operating gloves during dental procedures are:

- To protect patients from becoming infected with micro-organisms on the operator's hands.
- To protect the operator and staff from micro-organisms present in the patient's blood and saliva.

Intact hand skin provides good protection, but 40% of dentists have microlesions on the hands[1] which require added protection.

- To demonstrate to patients that the dental team are taking precautions to implement cross infection control.

Non-sterile latex gloves

Use non-sterile latex gloves for the following procedures:

- Examinations
- Routine restorative procedures
- Prosthetic and endodontic treatment
- Prophylaxis
- Radiography
- Laboratory work.

Choose a good-quality non-sterile latex glove; look for:

1. A glove which has been manufactured by the **double dip** process, using less irritating catalysing coagulants. These gloves have less pinholes than single dip gloves.
2. A glove which is powdered using **cornstarch** or **cetylpyridium chloride**. Talcum powder is a mineral material, which may cause irritation, and is not recommended.
3. A glove which conforms to statutory standards:
   - *USA* The American Society for Testing Materials (ASTM)[2] only specifies an acceptable leakage rate for sterile surgeon's gloves—*not* for non-sterile latex. The Food and Drug Administration (FDA) published the final rule relating to latex examination gloves on 12 December, 1990.[3] This ensures that latex examination gloves marketed in the USA are of a sufficiently high standard.
   - *UK* Non-sterile latex gloves must conform to the Department of Health (DOH) standard TSS/D/300/010/1 for non-sterile latex gloves (December 1990).
4. A glove which, according to published reports, has a low percentage of perforations prior to use.

Many brands of glove have been shown to be defective *prior* to use.[4-6]

Note: A simple inflation test that is available in the surgery, which demonstrates that a glove is not defective, may be useful. A glove defect detection test using fluoresin dye has also been described.[7]

Brands of glove recommended in the USA for use in dentistry, have been described.[8,9]

Single use versus re-use

Gloves may be satisfactorily cleansed of micro-organisms between patients. However, repeated use of one pair of gloves with disinfection between patients is not advisable for the following reasons:

- Exposure to disinfectants used to wash gloves after use causes defects and permeabiiity in gloves.[7]
- Chemicals used in routine dentistry damage gloves, e.g. Eugenol, Copalite varnish.[10]
- Gloves are damaged during use—studies have shown a high percentage of glove defects after performing dental procedures.[11–14]
- Prolonged use of gloves increases hand perspiration, which causes skin irritation.
- There is an increase in glove permeability to bacteria after use[15] and bacteria multiply beneath the glove material.[11]

After contact with a patient, gloves should be removed, the hands washed and disinfected, and new gloves applied before treating the next patient.

Recommendations for non-sterile glove use[16]

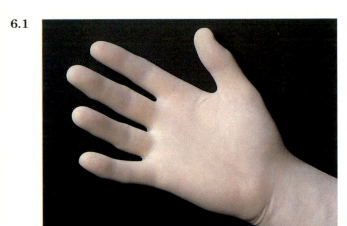

6.1 Choose a well-fitting glove. Avoid large-sized gloves with folds of rubber, especially around the finger ends.

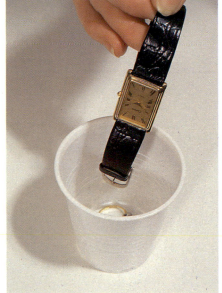

6.2 Remove rings and jewellery before gloving.

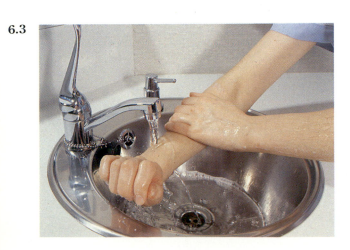

6.3 Wash, rinse, dry, and disinfect the hands before and after gloving.

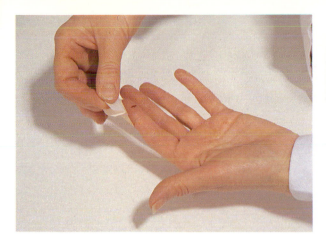

6.4 Cover cuts with a sterile waterproof dressing.

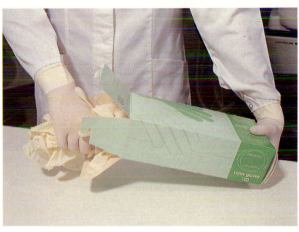

6.5 Draw gloves carefully from the container to avoid damage.

6.6

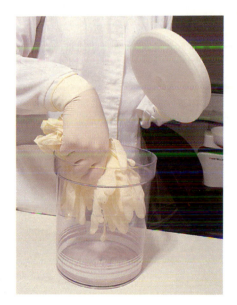

6.6 Place all gloves required for the clinical session in a safe container.

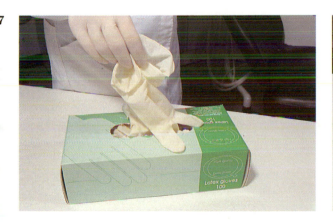

6.7 *Do not* pull gloves out of the top of the box, as it may cause glove damage.

6.8

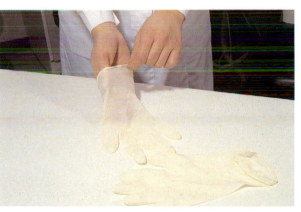

6.8 Slip one hand under the cuff and pull the glove carefully over the other hand.

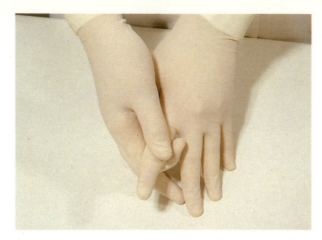

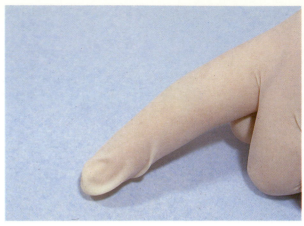

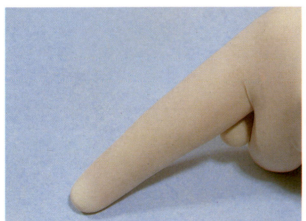

6.9–6.11 Pull each finger of the glove closely over each individual finger of the hand. Excess material at the finger tip (**6.10**) reduces tactile sensation and becomes easily caught up by instruments.

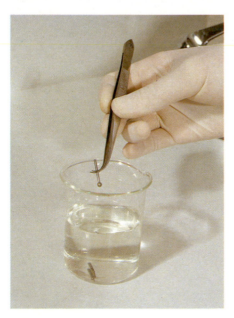

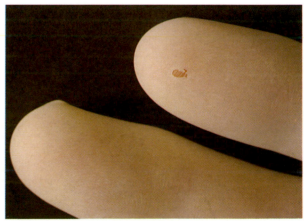

6.13 If a glove is punctured during use, discard it, wash and disinfect the hands, and put on a new pair of gloves. Change gloves after each treatment. Change gloves after prolonged use during treatment of the same patient, i.e. *after one hour*.

6.12 Handle sharp instruments carefully, to avoid glove puncture, e.g. burs should be picked up using tweezers.

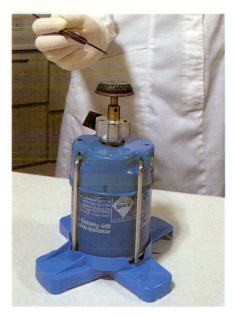

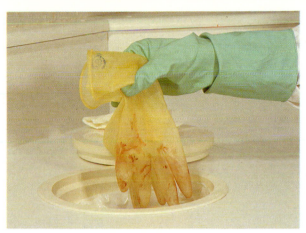

6.15 Gloves are potentially infected material, and careful disposal procedures should be followed.

6.14 Keep gloved hands away from naked flames.

Double gloving

Double gloving reduces the risk of puncture. A study has shown that the rate of puncture of the outer glove is 11%, while that of the inner glove is only 2% after use.[17]

Double gloving is of value either when the operator has dermatological conditions of the hand skin, or if patients are medically compromised.[13] The enhanced safety has to be balanced against the discomfort or reduced dexterity.

6.16

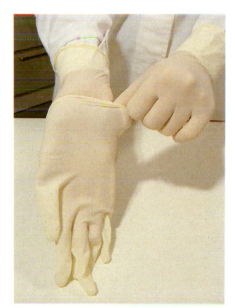

6.16 Double gloving.

Inflammability of glove material

Latex is highly inflammable and gloves may ignite on contact with a naked flame. If this occurs, removal of the burning glove may be difficult[18] and severe hand skin burns may occur (**6.17**).

An electric hot air blower (**6.18**) is now available which produces an even stream of hot air, at a con-trolled temperature. This is below the ignition point of latex, but hot enough to melt wax and heat instruments.

If a traditional Bunsen burner is used, dentists are advised to keep a dish of water close to the flame when gloves are worn.

6.17

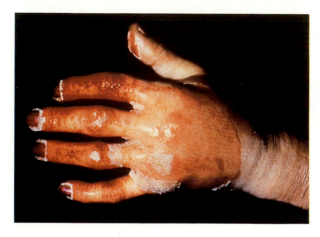

6.17 Hand damage from burning glove. (Courtesy Drs I.M. Brook and D.J. Lamb.)

6.18 The safe air heater. (Courtesy Drs I.M. Brook and D.J. Lamb.)

6.18

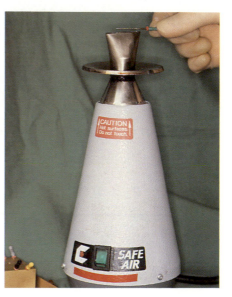

Latex gloves and polyvinylsiloxane impression material (addition cured silicone materials)

6.19

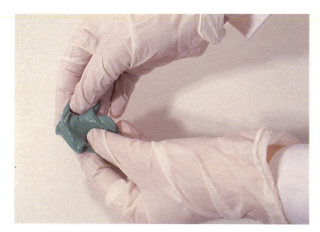

6.19 Overglove with vinyl gloves when mixing putty.

Many latex gloves contain accelerators such as **dithio-carbamate** products. Compounds of dithiocarbamate may inhibit the platinum catalyst in polyvinylsiloxane impression putty. When putty is mixed while wearing certain brands of latex gloves, the set of the putty is inhibited, or the bulk of the putty may set, but the surface remains tacky.[19] Overglove with vinyl gloves (**6.19**) when mixing such materials.

Degloved hands have also been found to be contaminated with dithiocarbamates, despite hand washing after glove removal.[20] Certain brands of gloves may *indirectly* inhibit the setting of polyvinylsiloxane material, due to the gloves depositing dithiocarbamates around the gingivae and the crown or bridge preparations. Gloves with a low content of accelerators, e.g. Travenol Ultraderm[19] or Biogel D, should be worn during crown and bridge preparation if poly-vinylsiloxane impression material is used.[19]

Note: A reagent which will detect the presence of thiocarbamate is currently being tested. This may enable the clinician to identify gloves which will not influence the set of polyvinylsiloxane impression material.[21]

Pulp testers and latex gloves

Unipolar pulp testers are used routinely in general dental practice. Such devices require the operator to complete the electrical circuit by touching the patient's lips or cheek. It has been found that gloved hands alter the wave form of the electrical current[22] and may prevent the registration of a vital response in a healthy tooth.[23]

To overcome this, it is recommended that the patient places the thumb and forefinger on the metal part of the pulp tester.[24] He is instructed to release the probe when he senses the flow of electrical energy (**6.20**).

A device supplied with some pulp testers (e.g. Analytic Technology pulp tester), connects the patient's lip to the pulp tester. This is useful when treating physically debilitated or handicapped patients.[24]

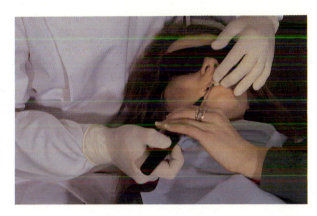

6.20

6.20 Recommended use of the pulp tester: the patient places the thumb and forefinger on the metal part.

Sterile latex gloves

Sterile latex gloves come in pairs contained in sealed packs (**6.21**). They are more expensive than nonsterile latex gloves.

Sterile latex gloves should be worn when performing either oral surgery, or periodontal surgery.

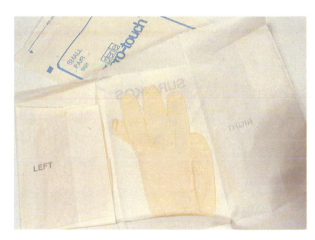

6.21

6.21 Sterile latex gloves.

Surgeon's gloves

Surgeon's gloves can be thicker than the latex gloves used in routine dentistry. They should be worn when carrying out either more extensive prolonged oral surgery, or implantology.

Orthodontist's gloves

Orthodontists have been shown to have the second highest incidence of hepatitis B among dental professionals.[25] The risk of glove puncture is high for orthodontists, who repeatedly handle wire bands and ligatures, although puncturing and tearing can be reduced by the use of elastomeric ligatures.[26]

One study has suggested that orthodontists consider a relatively puncture-resistant glove. This has greater thickness in the palm, a high stress area for ligature placement, and thinner material at the fingertips. The Aladan and Champag gloves meet these criteria.[26]

Vinyl gloves

Sterile and non-sterile vinyl gloves are available (**6.22**), however, these reduce tactile awareness.
  Vinyl gloves should be used if:

- The operator suffers from irritant contact dermatitis, or allergic contact dermatitis associated with latex gloves.
- The operator has to leave a patient during a procedure, e.g. to answer the telephone or to carry out an examination on another patient, vinyl gloves may be worn over latex gloves, and removed on returning to the patient (**6.23**).

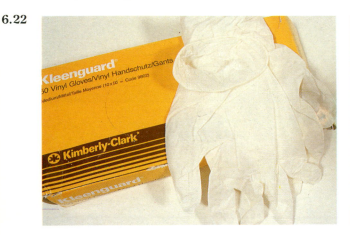

6.22   Vinyl gloves.

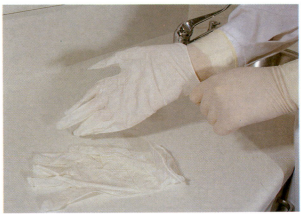

6.23   Overgloving.

General-purpose utility gloves

Thick, rubber utility gloves should always be worn when:

- Cleaning or packaging instruments (**6.24**).
- Disinfecting hard surfaces.
- Handling disinfectants and other irritant chemicals.
- Handling clinical waste.
- Performing general cleaning duties.

After use, the *gloved* hands should be washed with soap and water, thoroughly rinsed, and an alcohol-based disinfectant applied, e.g. Desderman (**6.25**).
  Each member of staff should have their own pair of rubber utility gloves, and should not use those belonging to another staff member. Utility gloves should be changed *weekly*, or when damaged.

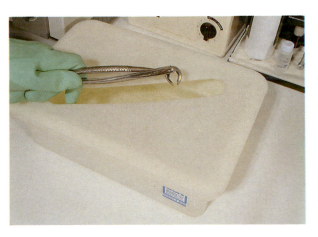

6.24   Wear utility gloves when handling sharp instruments.

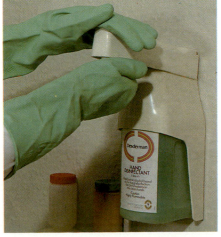

6.25   An alcohol-based disinfectant is applied to gloved hands.

Masks

Aerosols and splatter

Aerosols

Aerosols are airborne debris, smaller than 5 µm in diameter, that remain suspended in air, and can be aspirated into the bronchioles. Aerosols are generated by turbine handpieces, air/water syringes, and ultrasonic scalers. They may contain blood, but infection transmission by this means is considered unlikely. Infection transmission from aerosols is more likely if either the dental healthcare worker or the patient is suffering from influenza, the common cold, or other respiratory diseases.

Splatter

These are larger, sharp, blood-contaminated particles, generated by the turbine handpiece, ultrasonic scaler, and air/water syringe. They may damage the facial skin and eyes of the operator. Droplets of blood are also splattered over the face during dental procedures (**6.26**), and these may contact existing skin lesions or skin damaged by sharp, flying debris.

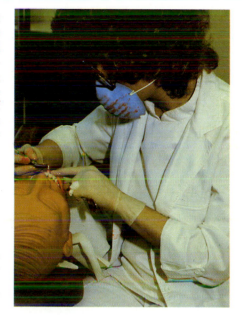

6.26

6.26 Splatter on masks and protective eyewear. (Courtesy Drs J. Molinari and J. Young).

Protection

The face and eyes must be protected when undertaking routine dental procedures. Masks protect the face from contaminated splatter and prevent inhalation of contaminated aerosols. It has been found that one of the primary factors determining mask life is the rate at which aerolised material soaks through (wicking).[27]

When choosing a face mask, it is essential that:

- It has a *bacterial filtration efficiency* (BFE) of 95% or more.
- It does not contact nostrils or lips.
- It has both high filtration of small particles and tolerable breathability.
- There is a close fit around the entire periphery.
- It does not cause fogging of eyeglasses.

The Clinical Research Associates (CRA)[28] tested 42 brands of facemask. They found that only 7 brands had a BFE of 95% or over. These were:

Magic Arch (Alpha Dental)
Dental Surgical (Alpha Dental)
Classic Surgical (Baxters)
Fluid Shield Surgical (Baxters)
High Filtration Isolation (Baxters)
Duckbill Surgical (Baxters)
Fog Free Surgical (Baxters)

A recent study has confirmed these findings.[27] Some of the conclusions reached in both these studies were that:

- Dental clinicians should consider alternatives to the traditional preformed cup design (**6.27**), which in most cases was found to have a much lower BFE.
- Before purchase of face masks, BFE test data on small particle (3.0–3.5 μm) aerosol filtration should be requested from dental manufacturers/distributors.
- The most efficient mask to be tested could only be worn for a maximum of one hour, in a high humidity environment.
- Face shields should not be worn without face masks.

- When a non-preformed mask becomes damp, it becomes not only uncomfortable, but also, if pathogens are present in the liquids soaking through the mask, potentially dangerous. A further study has shown that a mask becomes impregnated with micro-organisms after 20 minutes, becoming a source of contamination.[29]

A new mask that is available in the UK (Fluidshield), has an inner protective filter, which provides the mask with a BFE of 99% and resists penetration of contaminated fluids which collect on the outer mask layer (**6.28**). This mask also has an enclosed nosepiece, which is made of malleable aluminium and can be adapted to facial contours (**6.29**). This prevents 'fogging' of face shields or protective glasses.

6.27

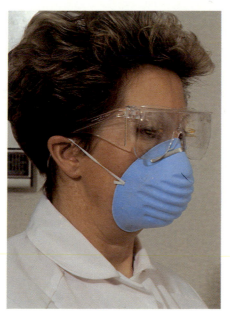

6.27   The preformed cup type mask.

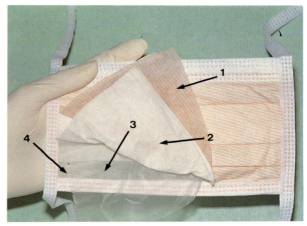

6.28   The Fluidshield mask showing four separate protective layers: 1 = outer facing; 2 = filter media; 3 = Loncet breathable film; 4 = inner facing.

6.29

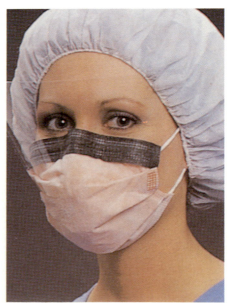

6.29   The nosepiece of the Fluidshield mask.

Eye Protection

Eyes may be damaged and infected[30,31] during dental procedures. Protective eyewear has been shown to reduce the likelihood of eye injury.[32]

Both dental healthcare workers and patients *must* wear eye protection during dental procedures.

Causes of eye damage

- Sharp particles projected at speed from the mouth when using the turbine handpiece, ultrasonic scaler, and air/water syringe may cause eye injury (**6.30**).
- Blood/saliva droplets may enter the operator's eyes and may transmit infection.
  e.g. Small amounts of blood containing the hepatitis B virus can cause infection if eye contact occurs.[33]

The spread of herpes type 1 virus may cause herpetic keratitis.[33]
Bacterial infection may occur (**6.31**).
- Injuries to the eyes of the patient can be caused by sharp instruments, especially when in the supine position.

6.31

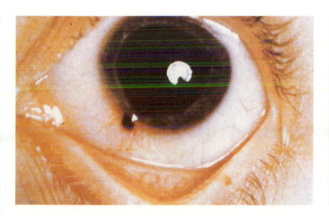

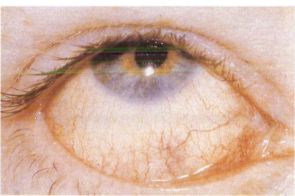

6.30 An eye injury caused during dental procedure. (Courtesy Dr M. V. Martin.)

6.31 Bacterial eye infections. (Courtesy Dr M. V. Martin.)

Types of eye protection

6.32

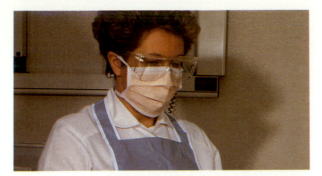

6.32 Protective glasses with side pieces. Some can be sterilised. Spectacles without side pieces are unsuitable. Coated safety glasses have the advantage of being fog and scratch resistant.

6.33

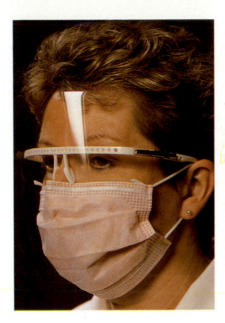

6.34

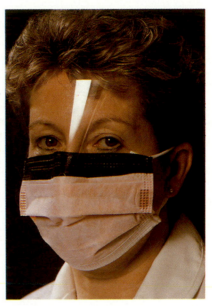

6.33 A chin-length face shield or visor protects the whole of the face. A mask should be worn under a face shield.

6.34 Disposable masks with a plastic face shield are available.

Fogging

Fogging of goggles or visors may be overcome by:

- Taping the top of the mask to the bridge of the nose with 3M hypoallergenic tape.

- Using a mask which may be closely adapted to the bridge of the nose.
- Using an antifogging liquid, e.g. Anti-mist marker.

Decontamination

Between patients, wash non-disposable protective eyewear with water and a detergent. Then, disinfect with a tuberculocidal hospital disinfectant, which does not damage the plastic or alter the ability of the eyewear to transmit light.[34] It should be noted that phenolics attack plastic. Always remove *all traces* of disinfectant from the protective eyewear by thorough rinsing with water.

Protective eyewear should not be handled with unprotected hands until it has been decontaminated.

Protective Clothing

To protect street clothes from contamination, wear a uniform or cover with a gown or coat.

Clothing should be made from synthetic material, with high collars and a minimum of seams, buttons, or buckles. Uniforms and gowns should be changed at least *daily*, and more often if they become visibly contaminated with blood.

When removing visibly contaminated clothing, fold the soiled area inside, being careful not to contaminate the hands. Put the soiled clothing into a commercial laundry or plastic bag. Send to a commercial laundry, or wash with hot water at 80°C for 10 minutes using a strong detergent, and bleach if possible.

Sleeves

Centers for Disease Control (CDC) and the American Dental Association (ADA) recommend *long-sleeved* uniforms. Tuck the bottoms of the sleeves into the gloves (**6.35**). Long sleeves protect the lower arms from blood splatter, especially if there is skin damage or wide-spread dermatitis on the arms.

Always remove protective clothing when leaving the surgery.

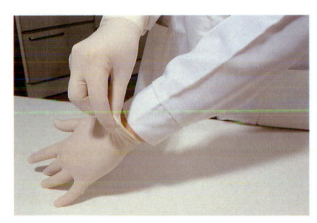

6.35

6.35 Tuck bottoms of the sleeves into the gloves.

Footwear

A pair of smooth, slip-on shoes should be kept exclusively for use in the surgery. These should be cleaned at the end of each clinical session.

Head covers

Head covers provide an effective barrier. They are recommended during invasive dental procedures which are likely to involve extensive blood splatter, e.g. extensive oral surgery.

Additional precautions

Masks, eye protection, and uniforms protect the dental healthcare worker from contaminated dental aerosols and splatter. There are other precautions which may be taken to *reduce* this risk:

- Pre-treatment tooth brushing,
- The use of a 2% (w/v) chlorhexidine pre-treatment mouthwash,
- High-volume aspiration,
- Correct use of rubber dam,
- Efficient air filtration and ventilation.

These are described in more detail in Chapter 7.

Avoiding Injuries

Handling sharp instruments

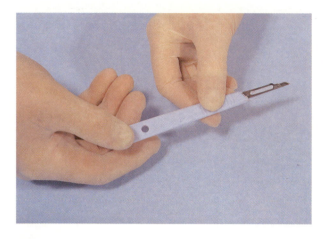

6.36 Point the sharp end of an instrument away from the hand.

Sharp items such as needles, scalpel blades, and other instruments should be considered potentially infective. They must always be handled with extreme caution, to prevent accidental injuries.

Take the following precautions when handling sharp instruments:

- Point the sharp end of an instrument away from the hand (passing from the right to left) (**6.36**).
- Pass syringes with the needles pointing away from anyone (**6.37**).
- Avoid handling large numbers of sharp instruments. Pick up instruments individually (**6.38**).
- Avoid hands contacting rotating instruments.
- Dispose of needles and other disposable sharp items immediately after use.
- Wear heavy utility gloves during clean-up.

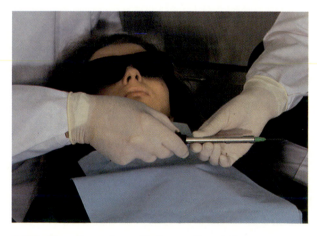

6.37 Pass the syringe with the needle pointing away.

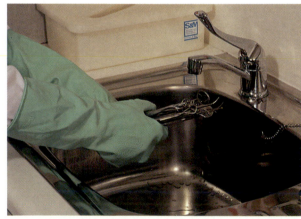

6.38 Avoid handling large numbers of sharp instruments.

Recapping dental syringes

- Do not attempt to remove an uncapped disposable needle from a syringe. This may cause a serious injury. Recap the needle using one of the **one-handed techniques** recommended (**6.39**).
- *Never* recap a needle using both hands (**6.40**), or by any other technique that involves moving the point of the needle toward any part of the body.
- The Septodont sharps container (**6.41**) incorporates an inbuilt device which assists in the safe removal of the needle from the body of the syringe.
- Between multiple injections given with a single needle, place the needle in a clean, *safe* position where it cannot be contaminated or cause accidental injury, or use a safe resheathing device (**6.42**).

In general:
Do not recap needles using two hands.
Do not bend, break or otherwise manipulate needles by hand.
Put used needles into a solid sharps container.

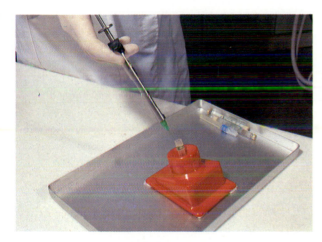

6.39 One-handed technique to recap a needle.

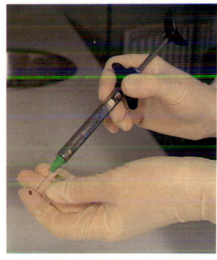

6.40

6.40 A needle should *never* be recapped using two hands.

6.41

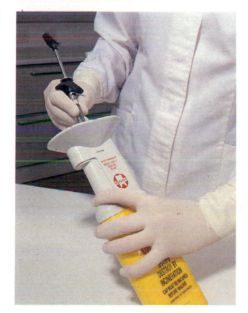

6.41 The Septodont sharps container.

6.42

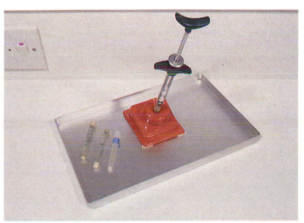

6.42 A resheathing device, between multiple injections.

The management of needlestick injuries

Every dental surgery should have a **written policy** for the management of injuries. This includes contamination of an open wound or of non-intact skin by blood or a mixture of blood and saliva.

The policy should include:

- The name of the person designated to receive a report of injuries and who is responsible for follow up.
- The name of the person who is designated to interview patients whose blood may be involved in an injury.
- A written log for recording injury (**6.43**) containing a detailed report of the accident.

All injuries that expose any member of the dental team to blood must be documented. All such information should be kept strictly confidential.

> **Log of injuries, including exposures to blood**
>
> Date of injury
> Person injured
> Cause of injury
> Patient name
> Description of events
> Witnesses
> Action taken
> Outcome
> Follow-up needed

6.43   Details to be recorded in the log of injuries.

Treatment of injuries

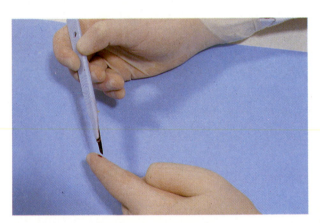

6.44   Gloved finger cut by scalpel.

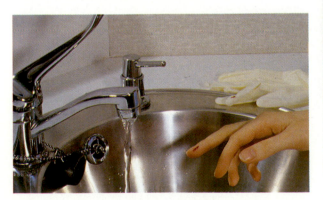

6.45   The glove is removed and the cut washed.

If an injury occurs which is caused by a blood-contaminated sharp instrument (**6.44**), wash the injury with soap and water (**6.45**). Do not scrub the wound. Encourage the wound to bleed, but do not suck the wound.

If the eyes are exposed, flood them with plain water (**6.46**).

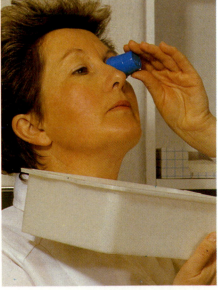

6.46   Plain water is used to irrigate the eyes.

Testing after injury

The injury should be reported to the member of the dental team who is responsible for follow-up. The risk from exposure to infected blood should be evaluated. If a risk is identified, laboratory tests and vaccination with immunoglobulin and hepatitis B vaccine may be necessary.

It is suggested that a sample of the dental health-care worker's blood should be tested immediately and the remainder stored. Further testing is then carried out at the end of the known incubation period. This procedure may be relevant to claims for industrial injury.

Laboratory tests might include testing for HIV and/or HBV and should be performed with appropriate counselling and follow-up if necessary. Testing should be performed in consultation with an appropriate physician.

Posters should be displayed in the surgery which explain *in detail* the steps to be taken following accidental exposure to blood (**6.47, 6.48**).

Hepatitis B virus postexposure management

IF	AND	THEN
The source individual is found positive for hepatitis B surface antigen (HBsAg).	The exposed worker has *not* been vaccinated against hepatitis B.	• The worker should receive the vaccine series for hepatitis B. • The worker should receive a single dose of hepatitis B immunoglobulin (HBIG) if it can be given within 7 days of exposure.
	The exposed worker *has* been vaccinated against hepatitis B.	The exposed worker should be tested for antibodies to HBsAg (anti-HBs), and given one dose of vaccine and one dose of HBIG if the antibody level in the worker's blood sample is <10 SRU by RIA, negative by EIA.
The source individual is found negative for HBsAg.	The exposed worker has *not* been vaccinated against hepatitis B.	The worker should be encouraged to receive hepatitis B vaccine.
	The exposed worker *has* been vaccinated against hepatitis B.	No further action is needed.
The source individual refuses testing or cannot be identified.	The exposed worker has *not* been vaccinated against hepatitis B.	• The worker should receive the hepatitis B series. • HBIG administration should be considered on an individual basis when the source individual is known or suspected to be at high risk of HBV infection.
	The exposed worker *has* been vaccinated against hepatitis B.	Management and treatment of the exposed worker should be individualised.

6.47 Management of persons exposed to blood: hepatitis B virus.

Human immunodeficiency virus postexposure management

IF	THEN	AND

The source individual has AIDS.
 	
OR
 	
The source individual is positive for HIV infection.
 	
OR
 	
The source individual refuses to be tested
	• The exposed worker should be counselled about the risk of infection.
	
	• The exposed worker should be evaluated clinically and serologically for evidence of HIV infection as soon as possible after the exposure.
	
	• The exposed worker should be advised to report and seek medical evaluation for any febrile illness that occurs within 12 weeks after the exposure.
	
	• The exposed worker should be advised to refrain from blood donation and to use appropriate protection during sexual intercourse during the follow-up period, especially the first 6–12 weeks after exposure.
		An exposed worker who tests negative initially should be retested
		  6 weeks,
		  12 weeks, and
		  6 months
		after exposure to determine whether transmission has occurred.

The source individual is tested and found seronegative.	Baseline testing of the exposed worker with follow-up testing 12 weeks later may be performed if desired by the worker or recommended by the worker's healthcare provider.	
The source individual cannot be identified.	Decisions regarding appropriate follow-up should be individualised. Serological testing should be done if the worker is concerned that HIV transmission has occurred.	

6.48 Management of persons exposed to blood: HIV.

Additional information—USA

Additional information is available in the following reprints from Morbidity and Mortality reports

• Recommended Infection Control Practices for Dentistry.
• Recommendations for Prevention of HIV Transmission in Healthcare Settings.
• Update: Universal Precautions for Prevention of Transmission of Human Immunodeficiency Virus, Hepatitis V Virus and Other Bloodborne Pathogens in Healthcare Settings.
• Update on Hepatitis B Prevention.

UK policy

Current policy in the UK is shown in **6.49**.

6.49

- Wash the wound or non-intact, exposed skin immediately under running tap water. Wash non-mucosal surfaces with soap.
- Record the accident.
- If not already vaccinated against HBV, give hepatitis B hyperimmune gamma-globulin *and* active immunisation. Accelerated vaccination at 0, 2, and 6 weeks, may be effective. The efficiency of immuno globulin has been questioned,[36] but it is generally said to be efficient.
- If already immunised, but more than 3 years before, give a **booster** of vaccine against HBV.
- If HIV is likely to be involved *expert* counselling of the wounded person (healthcare worker) and the patient is required. The patient and the healthcare worker should be advised to undergo a test for HIV. If the patient is HIV antibody-positive, the healthcare worker should avoid donating blood and should be tested after 3 or 6 months for HIV antibody. Antibodies usually appear within 3 months, but may not appear for up to 3 years. If a healthcare worker become HIV-positive, they and their family should be counselled and a specialist physician consulted.
- If an exposure of this type results in an illness, it needs to be reported formally by the employer under the Health and Safety (The reporting of injuries, diseases, and dangerous occurrences) Regulations (RIDDOR), 1985.
- The PHLS Communicable Disease Surveillance Centre (CDSC) and the Communicable Diseases (Scotland) Unit (CD(S)U) are conducting a national surveillance of accidental injury and other forms of contamination with HIV occurring in the UK.

6.49 Management of needlestick and sharps injuries (UK).[35]

Note: For more information consult:

Guidance for Clinical Healthcare Workers: Protection against Infection with HIV and Hepatitis Viruses. Recommendations of the Expert Advisory Group on AIDS. HMSO.

References

[1] Allen, A.L. and Organ, R. J. Occult blood under the fingernails, a mechanism for the spread of blood borne infections. *J. Am. Dent. Assoc.*, 1982;**105**:455–9.

[2] *American Standard Specification for Rubber Examination Gloves,* ASTMD 3578–87 (re-approved without change 1 Jan., 1982: 1–4) Philadelphia: American Society for Testing and Materials.

[3] FDA. *Medical Devices; Patient Examination and Surgeon's Gloves; Adulteration; Final Rule.* Federal Register, Department of Health and Human Services Food and Drug Administration, Part VI, 21:CFR Part 800.

[4] Burke, F. J. T., Alderson, J. J., Wilson, N. H. F. The incidence of holes in gloves supplied for routine use in clinical dental practice. *Dent. Practice*, 1988;**26**:14.

[5] Clinical Research Associates. Operating gloves, *Update* 1989; Vol. 13, Issue 1, January: 1–3.

[6] De Groot-Kosolcharoen, J. and Jones, J. M. Permeability of latex and vinyl gloves to water and blood. *Am. J. Inf. Control*, 1989;**17**(4):196–201.

[7] Bagg, J., Jenkins, S., Barker, G. R. A laboratory assessment of the antimicrobial effectiveness of glove washing and re-use in dental practice. *J. Hosp. Inf.*, 1990;**115**:73–82.

[8] Clinical Research Associates. *Newsletter,* 13/1, Jan. 1989.

[9] American Dental Association. *Clinical Products in Dentistry. A Desk Top Reference,* ADA.

[10] Ready, M. A., Schuster, G. S., Wilson, J. T., Hares, C. M. Effects of dental medicaments on examination glove permeability. *J. Prosth. Dent.*, 1989;**61**:499–503.

[11] Otis, L. L. and Cottone, J. A. Prevalence of perforations in disposable latex gloves during routine dental treatment. *J. Am. Dent. Assoc.*, 1989;**118**:321–4.

[12] Fell, M., Hopper, W., Williams, J. et al. Surgical glove failure rate. *Ann. R. Coll. Surg. Eng.*, 1989;**71**:7–10.

[13] Skaug, N. Micropunctures in rubber gloves used in oral surgery. *Int. J. Oral. Surg.*, 1976;**5**:220–5.

[14] Burke, F. J. T. and Wilson, N. H. F. The incidence of undiagnosed punctures in non-sterile gloves. *Br. Dent. J.*, 1990;**168**:67–71.

[15] Morgan, D. and Adams, D. Permeability studies on protective gloves used in dental practice. *Br. Dent. J.*, 1989;**166**:11–18.

[16] Burke, F. J. T. Non-sterile glove use, a review. *Am. J. Dent.*, 1989;**2**:255–61.

[17]Matta, H., Thompson, A. M., Rainey, J. B. Does two pair of gloves protect operating theatre staff from skin contamination? *Br. Med. J.,* 1988;**297**:597–8.

[18]Brook, I. M. and Lamb, D. J. A safe alternative to the gas flame. *Dent. Practice,* 1988;**26**:26.

[19]Kahn, R., Donovan, T., Chee, W. Interaction of gloves and rubber dam with poly (vinyl siloxane) impression material: A screening test. *Int. J. Prosthodont.,* 1989;**2**: 342–6.

[20]Reitz, C. D. and Clark, N. P. The setting time of vinyl polysiloxane and condensation silicone putties when mixed with gloved hands. *J. Am. Dent. Assoc.,* 1988;**116**:371–4.

[21]Burke, F. J. T., Lewis, H. G., Wilson, N. H. F. The effect of latex gloves on setting time of polyvinyl siloxane putty impression material. Letter to the Editor. *Br. Dent. J.,* 1989;**167**:158.

[22]Treasure, P. Capacitance effect of rubber gloves on electrical pulp testers. *Int. Endo. J.,* 1989;**22**:236–9.

[23]Booth, D. Q. and Kidd, E. A. M. Unipolar pulp testers and rubber gloves. *Br. Dent. J.,* 1988;**165**:254–5.

[24]Gailleteau, J. and Ludington, J. Using an electrical pulp tester with gloves, a simplified approach. *J. Endo.,* 1989; **15**:80–1.

[25]Starnbach, H. and Biddle, P. A pragmatic approach to asepsis in the orthodontic office. *Angle Orthod.,* 1980;**50**: 63–6.

[26]Cooley, R., McCourt, J., Barnwell, S. Evaluation of gloves for orthodontic use. *J. Clin. Orthod.,* 1989;**23**:30–4.

[27]Christenson, R. D., Robinson, R., Ploeger, B., Robinson, D., Leavitt, R. *Efficiency of 42 face masks and 2 face shields in preventing airborne particles.* (Unpublished data.)

[28]Clinical Research Associates Newsletter. Face masks. *Dental Clinical,* 1989;**13**:1–3.

[29]Craig, D. C. and Quale, A. A. The efficiency of face masks. *Br. Dent. J.,* 1985;**158**:87–90.

[30]Hales, R. A. Occular injuries sustained in the dental office. *Am. J. Ophthal.,* 1981;**70**:221–3.

[31]Palenik, C. J. Eye protection for the entire dental office. *J. Ind. Dent. Assoc.,* 1981;**60**:23–5.

[32]Roberts, H. T. J., Cass, A. E., Jagger, J. D. Occular injury and infection in dental practice. A survey and a review of the literature. *Br. Dent. J.,* 1991;**70**:20–2.

[33]Bond, W. W., Peterson, N. J., Favaro, M. S., Ebert, J. W., Maynard, J. E. Transmission of type B viral hepatitis B via eye inoculation of a chimpanzee. *J. Clin. Microbiol.,* 1982;**15**:533–4.

[34]Gleason, M. and Molinari, J. The stability of safety glasses during sterilisation and disinfection. *J. Am. Dent. Assoc.,* 1987;**115**:60–2.

[35]Scully, C., Cawson, R. A., Griffiths, M. *Occupational Hazards to Dental Staff.* British Dental Association, 1990, London.

[36]Iwarson, S. Post-exposure prophylaxis for hepatitis B: active or passive? *Lancet,* 1989;**2**:146–7.

7. Aseptic Technique

Limiting the Spread of Blood to Surfaces

During treatment and clean-up, blood and saliva-contaminated blood can be spread by anything that has been in the patient's mouth.[1] Blood may be spread around the operating zone either by contaminated gloved hands, or by splashes and splatter and, possibly, aerosols.

Contact with, and spread of, the patient's oral fluids was demonstrated during a series of procedures using the Columbia Dentoform mannequin. The oral cavity was coated with a solution of red dye to simulate saliva (**7.1**). Some of the common modes of fluid transfer were demonstrated (**7.2–7.10**).

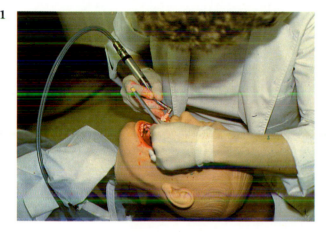

7.1 Dentoform mannequin.

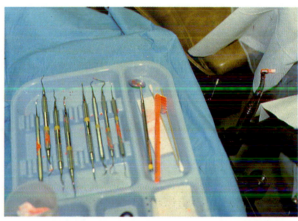

7.2 Instrument contamination.

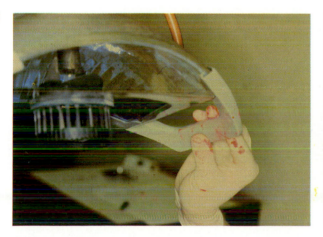

7.3 Contamination of the light handle.

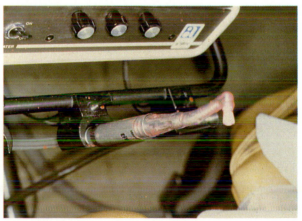

7.4 Handpiece contamination.

7.5

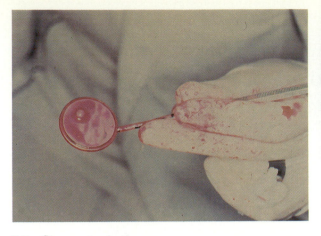

7.5 Glove contamination.

7

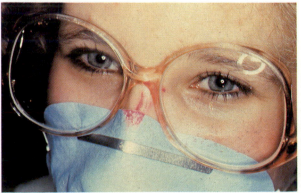

7.6 Contamination of the air/water syringe.

7.7

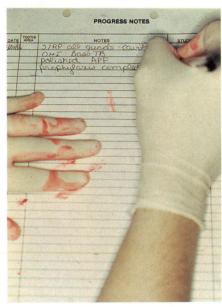

7.7 Contamination of the record card.

7.8

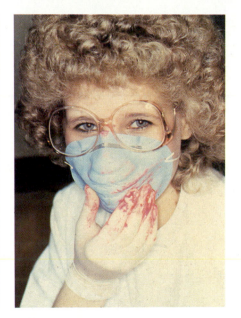

7.8 Face mask contamination.

7.9

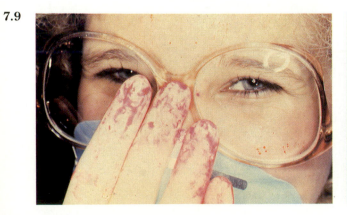

7.9 Touching protective eyewear.

7

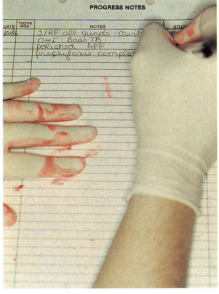

7.10 Contamination of protective eyewear.

(**7.1–7.10** Courtesy Drs J. Molinari and J. York and Detroit School of Dentistry.)

The dental team should use careful techniques, which prevent the *unnecessary* contamination of surfaces within the surgery. When this is not possible, such surfaces should be **covered** or **disinfected** after completion of the procedure.

Limiting surface contamination by good operating technique

Remove unnecessary items and unused or seldom used equipment from the operating area, leaving only necessary items on worktops. This reduces the number of items which could become contaminated, consequently making post-treatment clean-up easier.

Plan ahead, and anticipate items and instruments which will be required for the treatment of each patient. Instruments and materials which are overlooked are usually those obtained from packages in drawers or cupboards. During the dental procedure, this spreads pathogenic micro-organisms to surfaces that should remain clean and that are difficult to disinfect.[2]

Plan carefully and put out instruments, materials, and medication that will be required for each procedure. The use of unit-dose materials, e.g. prophylactic paste in a single-dose container, is important.

'Restriction zones'

These are areas to which contaminated items and instruments used for a dental procedure are confined. This prevents the spread of contamination from these instruments to wider areas around the operating zone.

Instruments, materials, and medications are placed in solid-based trays, positioned conveniently close to the dentist and nurse (**7.11–7.17**).

Anaesthetic tray

The anaesthetic tray (**7.11**) positioned near the dentist, contains:

- Disposable anaesthetic needle
- Local anaesthetic
- A recommended re-sheathing device.

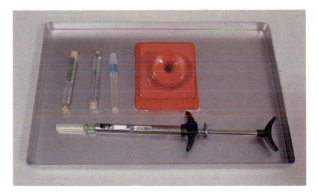

7.11

7.11 The anaesthetic tray.

Instrument tray

7.12

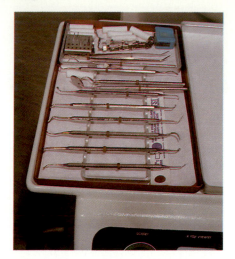

The instrument tray (**7.12**) is located on the bracket table. This may contain:

- Hand instruments
- Prophylactic polishing brush
- Rotary instruments required for the forthcoming procedure
- Triple syringe tip
- Matrix bands and holders
- Cotton wool materials
- Sterile bur changing tool.

7.12 The instrument tray.

Dentist's tray

7.13

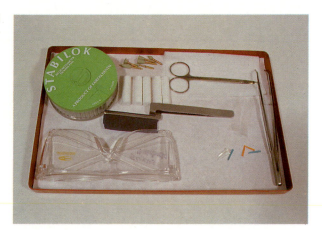

The 'dentist's' tray (**7.13**) is positioned near the dentist. This may contain:

- Matrix band strips
- Articulating paper
- Cotton wool materials
- Polishing stones
- Pins and wedges
- The dentist's protective eyewear
- Pair of sterile tweezers for transferring instruments and other items.

7.13 The dentist's tray.

Nurse's tray

7.14

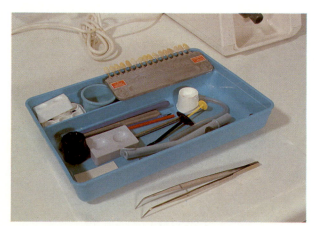

7.14 The nurse's tray.

The 'nurse's' tray (**7.14**) is positioned near the nurse. This may contain:

- Sterile amalgam carrier
- Autoclaved vacuum suction tip
- Disposable dappens pot
- Mixing spatulas
- Composite shade guide
- Disposable saliva ejector
- A small quantity of prophylactic polishing paste contained in a disposable dappens pot
- Unmixed cavity lining material
- The correct shade of composite, which is assessed (if required) before the procedure commences, is placed on the tray.

The unit-dose area

Unit-doses of materials are placed on a *covered* restricted area of the worktop, e.g. a unit-dose of impression material together with mixing utensils and impression syringe (**7.15**).

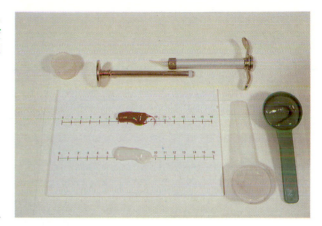

7.15 The unit-dose area.

The waste tray

An empty, solid-based 'waste' tray is placed near the dentist. Used, contaminated materials are placed onto this tray during the procedure (**7.16**).

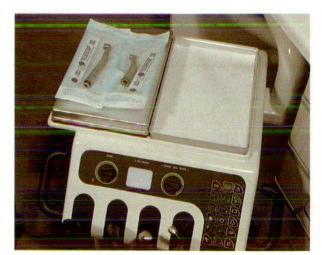

7.16

7.16 The waste tray.

Holding solution

A container filled with holding solution is placed near the dentist (**7.17**).

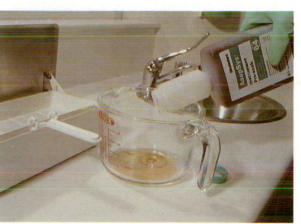

7.17

7.17 Holding solution.

Other considerations

Place the sterile handpieces onto the bracket table instrument tray at the start of the dental procedure. The bur block located on the instrument tray (**7.18**) should contain only the few burs required for the procedure. Additional sterile burs may be obtained from larger bur stands located near the dentist, but outside the operating zone. Obtain additional burs using sterile tweezers (**7.19**).

If instruments have to be taken from drawers or cupboards, the nurse should either overglove using a low-cost plastic glove (**7.20**), or use a tissue (**7.21**).

Preload mouthwash cups with a mouthwash tablet and store in a dispenser (**7.22**).

Locate the clinical notes and X-ray viewer outside the operating zone (**7.23**). The notes should be contained in a plastic wallet to prevent contamination.

Preparation is *very important*. Think ahead and place everything required for the dental procedure in pre-determined positions.

When items from the dentist's or nurse's tray are used, they are *not* returned to these trays, but are placed on the waste tray or in the holding solution. That is, **there is a one-way flow** (**7.24**), which minimises contamination of the trays and of the unused items on them. Cleaning and disinfection of the trays and remaining unused items is, therefore, kept to a minimum. When instruments or materials are taken from the dentist's or nurse's tray a pair of sterile forceps may be used to further reduce the spread of contamination.

7.18

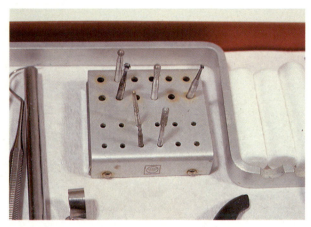

7.18   Bur block on the instrument tray.

7

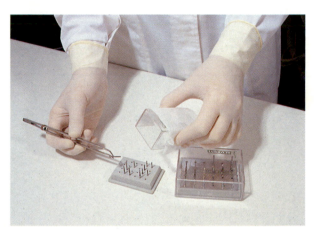

7.19   Larger bur block: remove the cover with a tissue and obtain burs using tweezers.

7.20

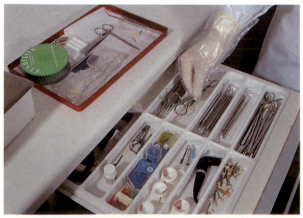

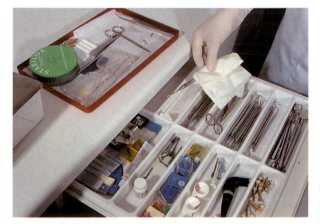

7.20, 7.21   To remove instruments from drawers during the procedure, either overglove with plastic gloves or use a tissue.

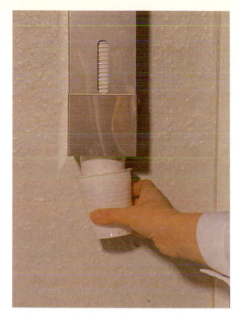

7.22

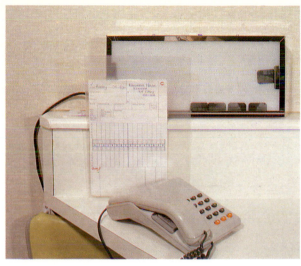

7.23 Clinical notes and X-ray viewer are located outside the operating zone.

7.22 Mouthwash cup dispenser.

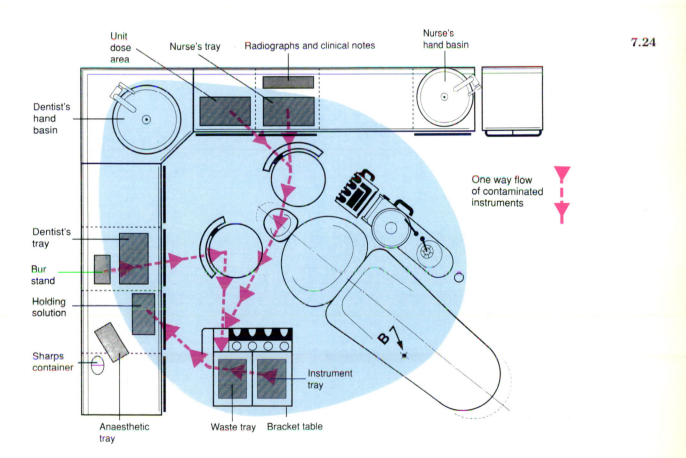

7.24

Unit dose area

Nurse's tray

Radiographs and clinical notes

Nurse's hand basin

Dentist's hand basin

One way flow of contaminated instruments

Dentist's tray

Bur stand

Holding solution

Sharps container

Anaesthetic tray

Waste tray

Bracket table

Instrument tray

7.24 Clean and dirty areas: showing the position of trays, the 'one-way' flow of contaminated instruments and other items, and the operating zone.

Covering or disinfecting environmental surfaces

There is evidence that, following dental procedures, surgery environmental surfaces are contaminated and pathogenic micro-organisms may survive on these surfaces for long periods of time.[3,4,5] It is difficult to prove that infection can be transmitted from surfaces in a clinical setting, but clinicians cannot ignore these studies or treat them lightly.[6]

To prevent contamination, surfaces in the operating zone should be either covered, or left uncovered and disinfected after treatment. The decision whether to cover or disinfect is determined by four factors:

- The likelihood of the surface becoming contaminated.
- The cost of disposable coverings.
- The time saved.
- Damage to equipment and surfaces by disinfectants.

A useful small booklet that describes cleaning and disinfecting surfaces is now available from Adec Ltd.

Covering surfaces

Surfaces *likely* to be contaminated can be covered while they are still clean.

Some surfaces such as light handles, hand-operated chair controls, suction hoses, chairs, and bracket tables are time-consuming and difficult to disinfect adequately.

Surfaces of some older dental units are damaged by the long-term application of disinfectants. Consider covering these surfaces.

Some examples of useful covers are illustrated (**7.25–7.28**). Use a disposable, waterproof covering, for example:

- Clear plastic wrap
- Aluminium foil
- Paper with impervious plastic backing
- Commercially available, polyethylene sheets and tubing

After each treatment:

- Remove the soiled covering while still gloved.
- Remove gloves and wash hands.
- Recover the surface with clean material before the next dental procedure.

This option may be expensive but has been found to be less time-consuming than surface disinfection.

7.25

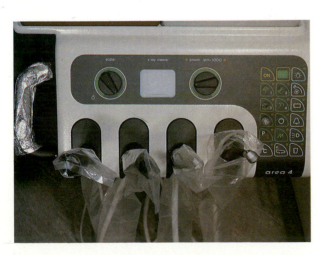

7.25 Covered air/water hoses and handles.

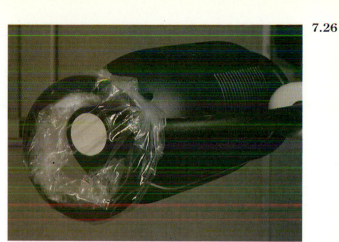

7.26 Covered light handles.

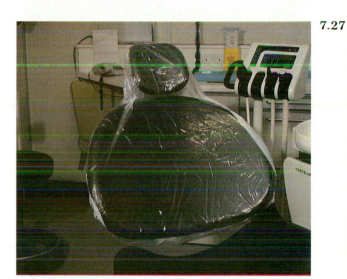

7.27 Chair cover.

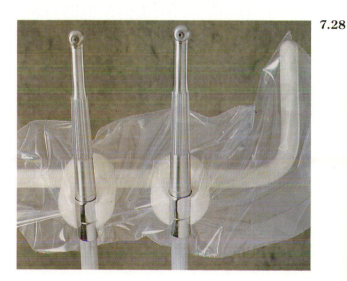

7.28 Bracket table cover.

Surface disinfection

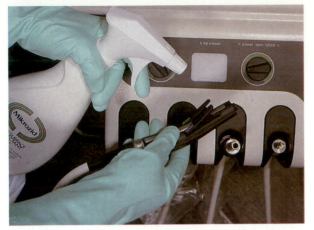

Environmental surfaces may become contaminated during a dental procedure. If these surfaces were not covered, they must be cleaned and disinfected.

Disinfect the surfaces in **7.29–7.37** after each dental procedure if trays have been used to restrict surface contamination.

Contamination may be reduced by handling certain surfaces using a tissue, e.g. the amalgam mixer (**7.38**); or by marking a small area on surfaces, e.g. bracket table handle (**7.39**). If only the marked surfaces are touched, these can be easily identified and disinfected.

7.29 The air/water syringe handle and tubing, and the handpiece outlet hoses.

7.30

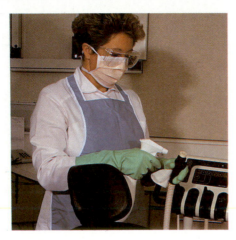

7.30 Ends of vacuum suction hoses.

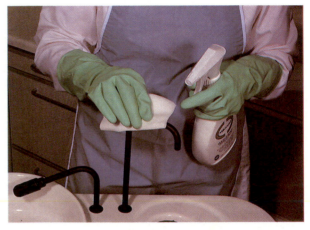

7.31 The spittoon and the area housing the mouthwash cup. Remember the outside of the spittoon.

7.32

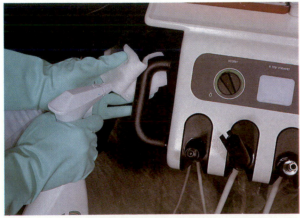

7.32 Operating handles and switches, including the operating light and bracket table handles and chair control switches.

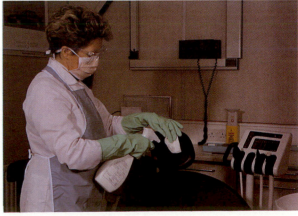

7.33 Chair arms and headrest. Remember the dentist's and nurse's chairs.

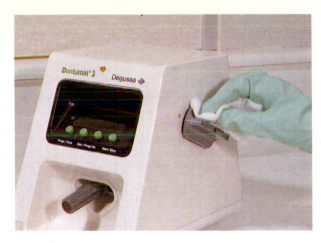

7.34 The amalgam mixer.

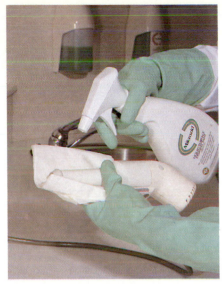

7.35 The light curing unit.

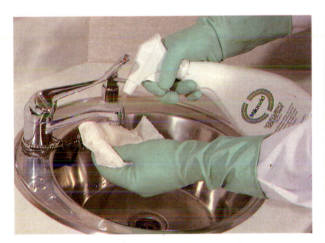

7.36 Sink areas—taps or levers.

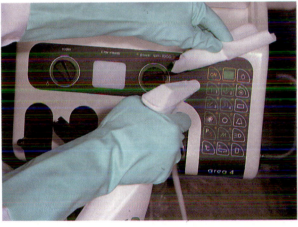
7.37

7.37 Unit control switches, which have been touched.

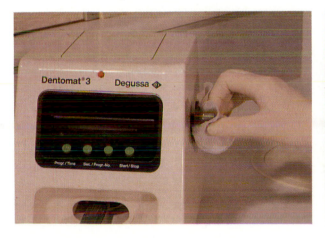

7.38 Handling the amalgam mixer using a tissue.

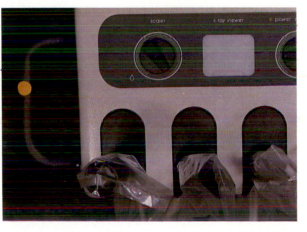
7.39

7.39 Small area marked on bracket table handle, to limit contamination.

Method of disinfection

7.40

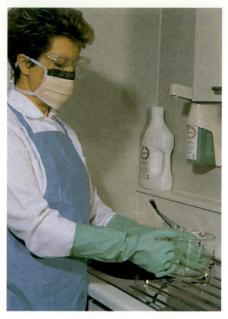

7.40 Wear heavy rubber gloves, a mask, protective eyewear, and a waterproof apron when disinfecting surgery surfaces.

When disinfecting the surgery surfaces, wear heavy rubber utility gloves, a mask, protective eyewear, and a waterproof apron, especially if a spray bottle is being used (**7.40**). Otherwise, prolonged use of disinfectants in this way may damage hand skin and eyes. The long-term detrimental effects of constant inhalation of aerosols containing disinfectants are unknown, and care must be taken.

The pre-cleaning stage

Surfaces must be cleaned before they are disinfected. Spray the surface with disinfectant (**7.41**) and wipe thoroughly (**7.42**) with a strong gauze sponge, e.g. cotton-filled gauze sponge by Healthco. The sponge should be renewed frequently if heavily soiled.

Note: Cotton has been implicated in the inhibition of the anti-microbial activity of iodophors. A recent research report[6] did not confirm this.

7.41

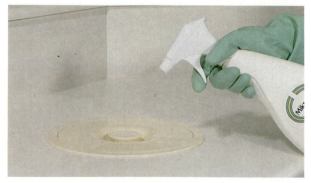

7.

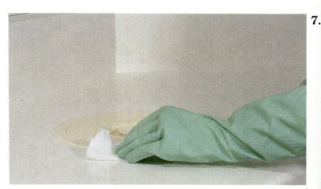

7.41, 7.42 The precleaning stage.

The disinfection stage

Respray (**7.43**) and leave the disinfectant on the surface for the recommended contact time (see Chapter 8). Wipe off residual disinfectant using a fresh paper towel.

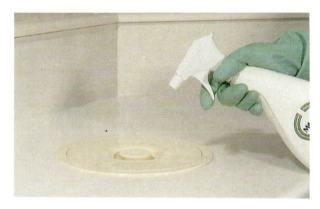

7.43   The disinfecting stage.

Recommended surface disinfectants

Solutions should be a **detergent** as well as a disinfectant.[7] Three surface disinfectants meet Environmental Protection Agency (EPA), American Dental Association (ADA), and Centers of Disease Control (CDC) requirements: sodium hypochlorite, iodophors, and combination synthetic phenolics.

The contact times and dilutions of a few products are shown in **Table 7.1**. These include ADA accepted products (as of January 1989); products have since been added to the list.

Table 7.1   Recommended surface disinfectants

Product	Dilution	Recommended contact time
Sodium hypochlorite 5.25% (Bleach)	1:10	10 min

Iodophors
  Biocide
  Surf-a-cide
	1:213	10 min

Combination synthetic phenolics
  Multicide
  Omni II
  Vitaphene
	1:32	10 min

All these materials have the disadvantage of leaving surfaces wet for *10 minutes*, which is inconvenient in a busy dental practice. Since 1978, the Council on Dental Therapeutics of the ADA has *not* accepted the use of alcohol as a disinfectant and there is substantial evidence supporting this approach.[8,9,10]

Glutaraldehyde products that are intended to be used as surface disinfectants contain only 0.25% (w/v) glutaraldehyde. However, they should be used with care, as repeated contact may damage the skin.[11] Do *not* use 2% (w/v) glutaraldehyde. The ADA does not recommend any glutaraldehyde products for use as surface disinfectants.

Surface disinfection using alcohol

Pre-cleaning is necessary to remove as much proteinaceous material (blood, saliva, and micro-organisms) as possible from the surface before application of a disinfectant. Precleaning is most effectively performed by the use of water-based solutions containing soap and detergent. Alcohols, or solutions containing a high alcohol concentration, are not as effective, as they cause denaturation and precipitation of proteins.[8] Recent research[6] indicates that products such as Citrace or Lysol sprays, containing 70% v/v denatured ethyl alcohol, were superior to 39 other surface disinfectants which were tested, including sodium hypochlorite, combination synthetic phenolics, and iodophors. This evidence is supported by recommendations issued by the Clinical Research Associates (CRA Newsletter, October 1989), who tested 72 environmental surface disinfectants. The CRA recommended disinfectants passing the CRA screen test, which indicates that they inactivated *Mycobacterium tuberculosis bovis*, and inactivated poliovirus I in 3 minutes or less.

Controversy still surrounds this topic. Some authorities recommend a single water-based product, which both cleans and disinfects. This has definite advantages, however such products leave surfaces wet for unacceptably long periods. The more realistic procedure in a busy dental practice is the use of a precleaner followed by an alcohol-based disinfectant, such as Lysol or Citrace (USA), Microzid or Hibispray (UK). These disinfectants act in 3 minutes, so surgery surfaces are dry before the next patient enters.

Author's recommendations

Disinfection of small surfaces between patients

Preclean, using the spray-wipe technique, with a recommended precleaning solution or water and detergent.

Spray with a product containing 70% alcohol, plus a low concentration of synthetic phenolic. Leave this solution on the surface for 3 minutes.

Disinfection of larger surfaces

Surfaces such as worktops or large areas of dental-unit surfaces are disinfected at the end of the day.

Preclean, using the spray-wipe technique, with an iodophor diluted 1:213.

Spray the iodophor onto the surface and leave wet, after wiping off any gross excess.

Note: It is not necessary to use a quick-acting and quick-drying solution in this situation. Alcohol-based disinfectants are expensive if used on such large areas. Reserve these for small areas between patients. Water-based disinfectants are cheaper to use on larger areas and have a residual disinfectant effect.

Other surface disinfectants

Surface disinfectants containing peroxygenated compounds are now available. One such product is Virkon which releases nascent oxygen and contains a detergent. These chemicals kill bacteria, viruses, and fungi, but their action on *Mycobacterium tuberculosis* has yet to be proven. They are very safe to use and are cost-effective. They have not yet been approved by the EPA.

Spillages

7.44

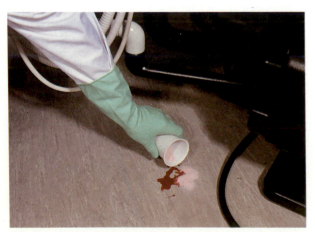

7.44 Using disinfectant granules to clean up a blood spill.

Gross spillages of blood or other contaminated fluids should be dealt with as follows:

- Cover the spillage with Virkon powder or Presept granules and leave for 3 minutes (**7.44**).
- Remove the residue using strong paper towels soaked in disinfectant (sodium hypochlorite or Virkon) and place these in a disposal bag.
- Repeat this procedure until all visible material is removed.
- Clean and disinfect the area using the spray/wipe/spray technique.

The spittoon waste filter

A spare, clean filter should be held in disinfectant solution. Between each patient, carefully remove the used filter from the spittoon (**7.45**), using a strong paper tissue, and take this to the sink. Pour liquid waste down a sink which is directly linked to a closed sewer (**7.46**). Solid waste must be put into a leak-proof bag with other solid waste. Carefully rinse the used filter and place into the disinfectant solution. Then fit the spare clean filter.

Filters become *very* contaminated. Remember to avoid a build-up of blood-contaminated material by *always* changing filters between dental procedures. Wear heavy utility gloves, eye protection, and a mask.

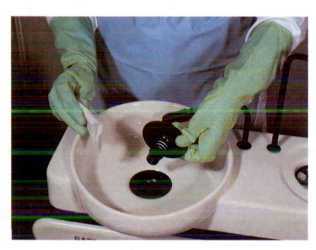

7.45 Remove the spittoon waste filter after each procedure, using a strong paper towel.

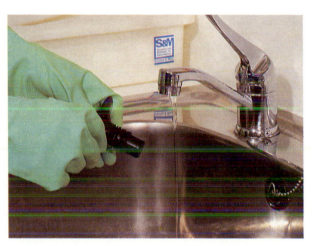

7.46 Carefully rinse the used filter.

Limiting Contaminated Aerosols and Splatter

During dental procedures and the clean-up period, aerosols, splatter of blood, and blood-contaminated saliva can be limited by:

- Pre-treatment tooth brushing and the use of a pre-treatment mouthwash.
- High-velocity aspiration.
- The use of a rubber dam, when possible.
- Efficient air filtration and ventilation.

Pre-operative tooth brushing and mouthwashes

7.47

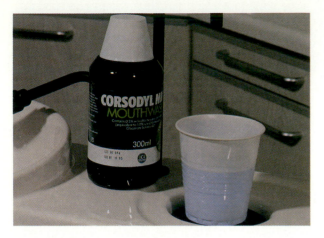

7.47 A 0.2% chlorhexidine mouthwash.

Instruct the patient to brush the teeth shortly before attending for treatment. Provide a 0.2% chlorhexidine mouthwash (**7.47**). This is used by the patient for *2 minutes* immediately before treatment begins.

These precautions have been found to reduce the concentration of bacteria in dental aerosols,[12,13,14] however, they have *minimal* effect on the reduction of cross infection risk from dental splatter.[12]

High-velocity aspiration

7.48

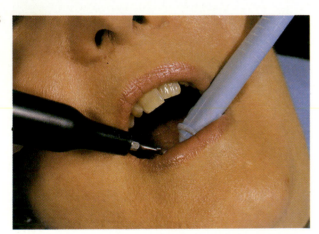

7.48 Use of high-velocity aspiration.

It has been shown that when high-velocity aspiration (**7.48**) is correctly used with the turbine handpiece, the air/water syringe, or the ultrasonic scaler, contamination from aerosols is reduced.[14] The suction must exhaust externally, *not* into the room.

Decontamination of high-velocity aspiration equipment

High-velocity aspirators become very contaminated. Effective disinfection of high-velocity aspiration equipment primarily provides protection for the people who clean and maintain the unit.

The daily routine
This should be carefully implemented.

At the end of the day, aspirate 1 litre of non-corrosive, non-foaming disinfectant, e.g. AC20 (a non-foaming, low-concentration, stable, glutaraldehyde-based disinfectant)[15] into *each* aspirator tube (**7.49**). Thoroughly clean and disinfect the outer surface of the tubes with an iodophor surface disinfectant.

Certain dental units have aspirator tubes which can be detached. At the end of the day, detach these tubes and soak in an EPA disinfectant/sterilant solution overnight (**7.50**).

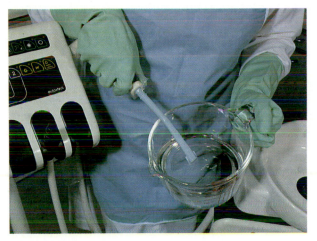

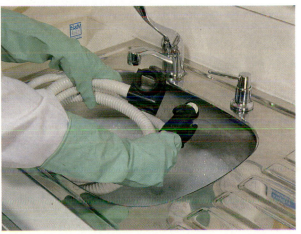

7.49 Aspirate non-foaming disinfectant into each aspirator tube.

7.50 Soak detachable aspirator tubes overnight in a liquid disinfectant.

Mobile aspirators

Mobile aspiration systems contain a bottle which is one-third filled with disinfectant prior to use. All aspirated material is mixed with disinfectant *in situ*.

Do not allow aspirator bottles to overfill. Dispose of the bottle contents down a drain or a sink with a direct link to a sewerage system.

The suction trap

This should be cleaned and disinfected weekly. Daily disinfection of aspirator tubes can substantially reduce the microbial flora associated with solid-waste filter traps.[16] In addition, empty the suction trap *after* disinfecting the suction system.

Remove the suction trap and, being careful not to spill or splash, pour the liquid into a drain linked to a closed sewerage system (**7.51**). Put the solids into a leakproof bag with other solid clinical waste. Soak the suction trap in EPA disinfectant/sterilant overnight.

Always wear heavy rubber utility gloves, protective eyewear, and a mask when completing these routines.

Disposable solid waste filter traps are available (Dispos-a-trap, Pinnacle Dental, USA).

Some units have systems permitting safe and minimal cleaning (see Chapter 11).

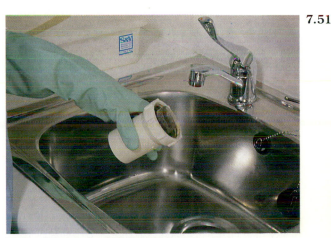

7.51 Pouring the liquid waste from a suction trap into a sink connected to a closed sewerage system.

The rubber dam

7.52

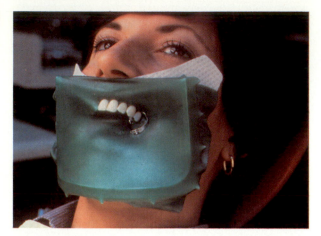

7.52 The rubber dam.

A rubber dam (**7.52**) should be used whenever possible during dental procedures. It has been found that there is a *significant* reduction of pathogenic micro-organisms generated in aerosols and splatter, if a rubber dam is used with the turbine handpiece, air/water syringe, or the ultrasonic scaler (**7.53–7.55**).[17,18]

7.53   **7.54**

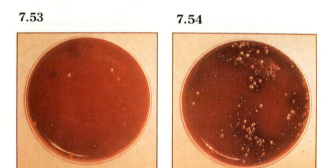

7.53, 7.54 Microbial samples collected on petri dishes placed near the patient's mouth during preparation and placement of restorations. With dam (**7.53**), 32 CFUs; without dam (**7.54**), 251 CFUs.

7.55

Latest Infection Control Data

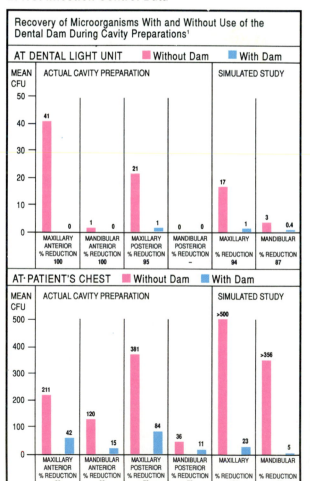

Recovery of Microorganisms With and Without Use of the Dental Dam During Cavity Preparations[1]

AT DENTAL LIGHT UNIT ■ Without Dam ■ With Dam

ACTUAL CAVITY PREPARATION

MEAN CFU	MAXILLARY ANTERIOR	MANDIBULAR ANTERIOR	MAXILLARY POSTERIOR	MANDIBULAR POSTERIOR	MAXILLARY (SIMULATED)	MANDIBULAR (SIMULATED)
Without Dam	41	1	21	0	17	3
With Dam	0	0	1	0	1	0.4
% REDUCTION	100	100	95	–	94	87

AT PATIENT'S CHEST ■ Without Dam ■ With Dam

ACTUAL CAVITY PREPARATION   *SIMULATED STUDY*

MEAN CFU	MAXILLARY ANTERIOR	MANDIBULAR ANTERIOR	MAXILLARY POSTERIOR	MANDIBULAR POSTERIOR	MAXILLARY (SIMULATED)	MANDIBULAR (SIMULATED)
Without Dam	211	120	381	36	>500	>356
With Dam	42	15	84	11	23	5
% REDUCTION	80	88	78	70	>95	>99

7.55 Data indicating reduction in airborne contamination if a rubber dam is used during actual cavity preparation and a simulated study.

Ventilation and air filtration

Laminar air flow and ventilation

This method reduces possible contamination from aerosols. It involves ventilating a room in such a way as to create a down draught through a large filter in the ceiling. By filtering recirculated air and by introducing a substantial proportion of fresh air in each air change this will substantially reduce residual contaminated aerosol.[19]

A simple air-circulation and filtration system may be used, e.g. a small window air-conditioning unit (**7.56**) and an exit-grille low down on a door in the opposite wall.[19]

It has been found that portable electrostatic precipitation units (**7.57**) are useful in reducing the level of aerosol contamination in a surgery.[13]

The filters should be changed frequently, wearing rubber utility gloves. Place the filter in a strong plastic bag, which is then sealed.

7.56

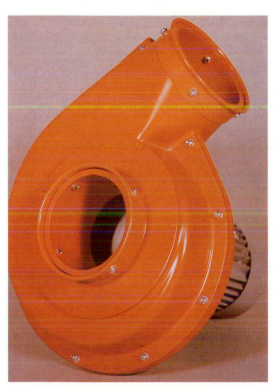

7.56   An extraction fan suitable for a dental office.

7.57

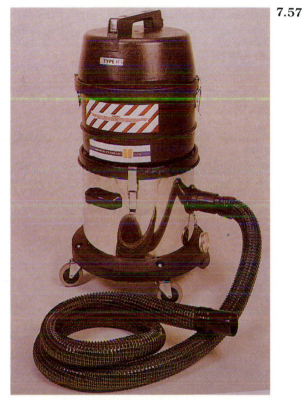

7.57   A free-standing electrostatic precipitation unit.

Disposables

In an ideal world, everything within reason that is used in dentistry should be disposable. Dental supply companies advertise a vast range of disposable products, some of which would prove very expensive over a period of time to the dental practitioner.

Two rules determine the choice of disposable from non-disposable:

- If an instrument or item cannot be satisfactorily sterilised or disinfected, as appropriate, then choose a **disposable alternative**.
- If an instrument or item can be appropriately sterilised or disinfected quickly, efficiently, and with *minimal* damage, do not use the disposable alternative unless it is very cheap and of similar quality.

There are certain items used in dentistry which it is suggested may be disposable. A few are listed.

Anaesthetic needles and cartridges (7.58): it is *mandatory* that these items are never re-used as they cannot be satisfactorily sterilised.

Mouthwash cups/beakers (7.59) become very contaminated and plastic disposable beakers are available at a low cost. Plastic cups are pre-loaded with mouthwash tablets, and are placed in a wall-mounted dispenser.

Saliva ejector tips (7.60): these are difficult to clean and sterilise and low-cost disposable tips should be used.

Intra-oral radiograph holders (7.61): simple, low-cost disposable holders are recommended.

The patient's protective bib (7.62) becomes splattered with blood and debris during dental procedures and is difficult to clean and disinfect. Disposable bibs are available and these should have an upper paper porous layer and a lower non-porous layer.

Surgical masks have been described in Chapter 6.

Operating gloves have been described in Chapter 6.

Disposable impression trays (7.63) are now widely used in dentistry. The handles can be detached and autoclaved. If metal trays are used, they should be thoroughly cleaned and autoclaved before they are used again.

Prophylactic polishing cups and brushes are highly contaminated after use (**7.64**). Brushes and prophylactic polishing cups cannot be effectively decontaminated and sterilised without damage and should be regarded as disposable.

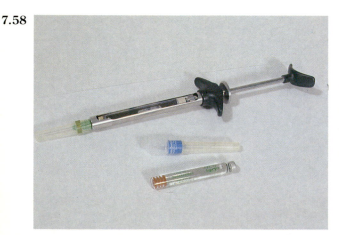

7.58 Anaesthetic needles and cartridges.

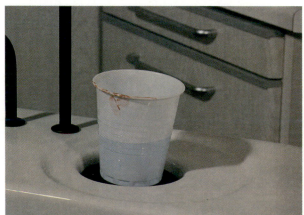

7.59 Contamination on a mouthwash beaker.

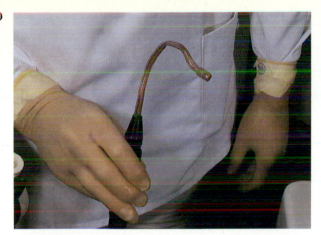

7.60 Saliva ejector tips.

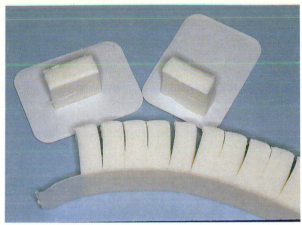

7.61 Intra-oral radiograph holders.

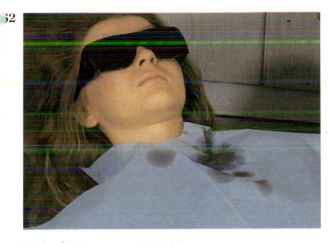

7.62 Splatter on a patient's bib.

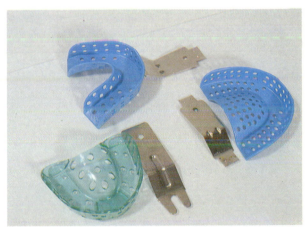

7.63 Disposable impression trays.

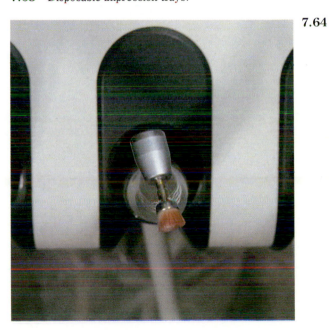

7.64 Contaminated brush.

General Cleaning of Surgery and Office

General cleaning of the office and surgeries should be carried out to a very high standard by cleaning staff. They should be made aware of danger areas in the surgery. Cleaning of cabinets, the dental unit, and other equipment should be undertaken by the dental surgery staff. Clinical waste disposal should be undertaken by dental surgery staff.

The following routine is suggested for treatment and non-treatment areas:

Non-treatment areas (e.g. reception): *Daily*—dust and wipe with disinfectant.

Patient treatment areas:

- *Monthly*—clean and disinfect drawers and cabinets with a long-acting disinfectant, e.g. iodophore. Bulk storage areas should be checked and cleaned every 3 months.
- *Weekly*—disinfect those areas of hard surfaces which are not disinfected daily, e.g. backs and sides of cabinets.
- *Daily*—clean and disinfect all worktops, cabinet fronts (especially around the operating zone), the surfaces of the dental unit and chair, and X-ray apparatus. Wash floors using a disinfectant/detergent solution. Disinfect the sink and spittoon drains using sodium hypochlorite.

Note: **Floor coverings** in a surgery should be hard, sealed, and continuous with no cracks. Carpets should be avoided in the treatment area, but if used nearby, should be low-pile, synthetic kitchen type which are capable of disinfection.

Handling Biopsy Specimens and Extracted Teeth

Biopsy and microbiological specimens

Use a sturdy container which will not leak or break (**7.65**). Seal the lid securely. Do not contaminate the outside of the container with blood when collecting the specimen.

If the outside of the container is visibly soiled, clean it first, then disinfect it using an EPA-registered tuberculocidal 'hospital disinfectant'. Be careful not to allow any disinfectant into the container or onto the specimen itself.

If specimens are to be sent by post, *strict* adherence to regulations pertaining to transport of infective material is essential. Attach a hazard warning label to containers of biopsy or microbiological specimens, this may contain the words 'pathological specimen'. Microbiological specimens should be securely bagged, with the request form enclosed separately to prevent contamination (**7.66**).[20]

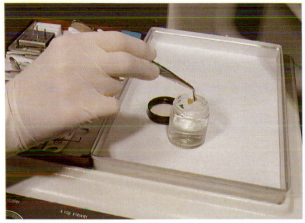

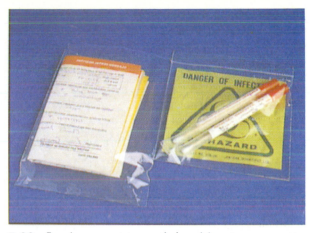

7.65   A solid container suitable for a biopsy specimen.

7.66   Specimens sent to a pathology laboratory are separate from the instructions. (Courtesy Dr L. P. Samaranayake and *Dental Update*.)

Extracted teeth

Wear gloves to handle extracted teeth. Place the teeth into a self-seal, leakproof bag and dispose of as infective solid waste, as described in Chapter 12.

References

[1]Molinari, J. A. and York, J. Cross contamination visualisation. *C. D. A. Journ.*, 1987;**15(9)**:12–16.

[2]Rothwell, P. S. and Dinsdale, R. C. W. Cross infection control in dentistry. The practicability of the zone system. *Br. Dent. J.*, 1988;**165**:185–7.

[3]Piazza, M., Guadaynino, V., Picciotto, L., Borgia, G., Nappa, S. Contamination by hepatitis B surface antigen in dental surgeries. *Br. Med. J.*, 1987;**295**:473–4.

[4]Thomas, L., Sydiskis, R., DeVore, D., Krywolap, G. Survival of herpes simplex virus and other selected microorganisms on patients' charts: potential source of infection. *J. Am. Dent. Assoc.*, 1985;**11**:461–4.

[5]Autio, K. L., Rosen, S., Reynolds, N. J., Bright, J. S. Studies on cross contamination in the dental clinic. *J. Am. Dent. Assoc.*, 1980;**100**:358–61.

[6]Christenson, R., Robinson, R., Robinson, D., Ploeger, B., Leavitt, R., Bodily, H. Antimicrobial activity of environmental surface disinfectants in the absence and presence of bioburden. *J. Am. Dent. Assoc.*, 1989;**119**:493–505.

[7]OSAP Position Paper 7-002. *Surface Disinfection Procedures for Disinfecting Surfaces and Equipment.* Denver: Office Sterilisation and Asepsis Procedures Research Foundation, 1988.

[8]Molinari, J., Merchant, V., Gleason, M. Controversies in infection control. *Dental Clinics of North America,* 1990; **34**: 55–69.

[9]Molinari, J., Gleason, M., Cottone, J., Barrett, E. Cleaning and disinfectant properties of dental surface disinfectants. *J. Am. Dent. Assoc.*1988;**117**:179–82.

[10]Molinari, J., Gleason, M., Cottone, J., Barrett, E. Comparison of dental surface disinfectants. *General Dent.*, 1987; **35**:171–5.

[11]Hess, J., Molinari, J. A., Gleason, M. J., Radecki, C. Epithelial toxicity of dental disinfectants. *Am. J. Dent.*, 1991;**4**:51–6.

[12]Wyler, D., Miller, R., Micik, R. Efficiency of a self administered pre-operative oral hygiene procedure in reducing the concentration of bacteria in aerosols generated during dental procedures. *J. Dent. Res.*, 1971;**50**:509–13.

[13]Muir, K. F., Ross, P. W., MacPhee, I. T., Holbrook, W. P. Reduction of microbial contamination from ultrasonic scalers. *Br. Dent. J.*, 1978;**145**:76–8.

[14]Worrall, S. F., Knibbs, P. J., Glenwright, H. D. Methods of reducing bacterial contamination of the atmosphere arising from use of an air polisher. *Br. Dent. J.*, 1987;**163**: 118–19.

[15]Gorman, S. P. and Scott, E. M. A comparative evaluation of dental aspirator cleansing and disinfectant solutions. *Br. Dent. J.*, 1985;**158**:13–16.

[16]Merchant, V. and Molinari, J. Evacuation system lines and solid waste filter traps associated flora and infection control. *General Dent.*, 1990;**38**:189–93.

[17]Cochran, M., Miller, C., Sheldrake, M. The efficacy of the rubber dam as a barrier to the spread of microorganisms during dental treatment. *J. Am. Dent. Assoc.*, 1989;**119**:141–4.

[18]Samaranayake, L. P., Reid, J., Evans, D. The efficacy of rubber dam isolation in reducing atmospheric bacterial contamination. *J. Dent. for Children*, 1989;**56**:442–4.

[19]Grundy, J. R. Hazards from aerosols. *Dental Update*, 1979;**6(7)**:483–9.

[20]Samaranayake, L. P. On the wastage of microbiological samples in clinical practice. *Dent. Update*, 1987;**14**:53–61.

8. Disinfection and Disinfectants

Disinfectants are used in dentistry as: immersion disinfectants; hard surface disinfectants; and disinfectants used in the dental unit water supply, drains, and high-velocity aspirators.

EPA and ADA Registration

Semi-critical items damaged by heat, or non-critical items are decontaminated using specific disinfectants regulated by United States federal law.

Under the Federal Insecticide, Fungicide and Rodenticide Act (FIFR Act, amended 1978) the USA Environmental Protection Agency (EPA) registers all chemicals used as **disinfectants** and **sterilants** on **inanimate** objects. The EPA reviews the efficiency and toxicity of these, and each approved product is given an EPA registration number which must be shown on the product label.

The American Dental Association (ADA) Council on Dental Therapeutics also evaluates each product and *recommends* only those that are suitable, efficient, and safe. An ADA acceptance programme does not have the same legal implications as the FIFR Act, but it is important to confirm that a product is ADA approved. In general terms, when choosing a disinfectant make sure that it has an EPA Agency Number displayed on the product label, and that it has an ADA seal of acceptance.

Federal law dictates that the Food and Drug Administration (FDA) should register all disinfectants used on the human body and a National Drug Commission (NDC) number is issued to each product that satisfactorily completes the FDA registration process. These regulations apply to disinfectants used for hand washing.

The EPA puts chemicals into four classes of use:

1. **Disinfectants/sterilants:** may be used for sterilisation or high-level disinfection, depending on the contact time.

2. **Hospital disinfectants with tuberculocidal activity:** are used to achieve intermediate disinfection.

3. **Non-tuberculocidal hospital disinfectants:** are used to achieve low-level disinfection.

4. **Sanitisers.**

Chemicals from Groups 1 and 2 are usually used in dentistry. The names of the EPA classes of chemicals are controlled by law. The manufacturer of a disinfectant cannot use these terms without EPA approval. They appear on the label of any chemical registered with the EPA.

Reading the labels

Any chemical disinfectant used should have a label that shows the EPA classification, the EPA registration and establishment numbers, and the directions for use and disposal. The label details are important and should be checked before using a disinfectant.

Additional label information

If the words disinfectant/sterilant and sporicidal are on the label, the chemical can be used for either sterilisation or high-level disinfection. The same concentration of chemical is used for both processes, but a longer contact time, as given on the label, is used for sterilisation.

If a chemical is to be used for intermediate-level disinfection, look for the terms tuberculocidal and hospital disinfectant.

A chemical which is used for low-level disinfection has the term hospital disinfectant, but the label does not indicate that it is tuberculocidal. In fact, the label might state that it may not produce thorough disinfection in the presence of *M. tuberculosis bovis*. This group of disinfectants will only inactivate certain vegetative bacteria and lipid viruses in the absence of gross organic soil.

Disinfectants Used in Dentistry

Aldehydes

Formaldehyde

Formaldehyde solutions have a pungent, suffocating odour, and an irritating effect on skin and mucous membranes. These solutions are not recommended for routine use in dentistry.

Glutaraldehyde

Recommended by the EPA for the *immersion* of instruments using a 2% w/v solution. These solutions achieve sterilisation or high-level disinfection depending on the immersion time shown on the label.

Solutions available

Glutaraldehydes are available as neutral solutions (pH range 7.0 to 7.5), alkaline solutions (pH range 7.0 to 8.5), and acidic solutions (pH range 4.0 to 6.5). Most products in the neutral and alkaline range must be activated before use by adding an appropriate buffer. Unused solutions remain active for 14–30 days depending on the preparation. This is known as the **use life** and should be shown on the label. The **shelf life** is the length of time the disinfectant may be safely stored in its original state and this information should also be available on the product label (this is now an EPA regulation).

Most products in the acidic pH range need not be activated prior to use and have a shelf life of two years or more. Follow the label directions for the appropriate use of these products.

Reuse of glutaraldehydes

Activated glutaraldehyde is EPA approved for reuse. Manufacturers must submit data to EPA substantiating claims for prolonged reuse (over one day) of prepared solutions and the EPA requires manufacturers to state the reuse time on the product label.

Test kits (**8.1**) are available which indicate the concentration of active glutaraldehyde remaining in the disinfectant solution under reuse conditions. These kits do not measure biocidal activity and some have been found to be unreliable.[1,2] Products should not be reused beyond the number of days or the number of use cycles specified on the product label. If the solution is routinely used, it may be better to make up a fresh solution earlier than the reuse date.

Adverse reactions and precautions

Undiluted solutions can cause irritation of the eyes and skin.[3] Contact should be avoided. Utility gloves, a mask, and eye protection *must always* be worn when mixing or handling glutaraldehyde. Solutions should be used only in an area with good ventilation, and containers must be covered. This group of disinfectants is not recommended for use on surfaces.

8.1

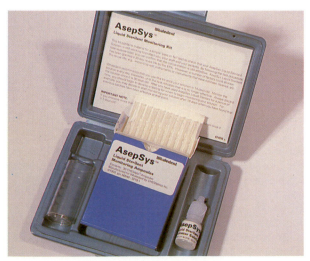

8.1 Test kit for use on disinfectant solutions.

Glutaraldehyde—phenate solutions

Glutaraldehyde phenate is an alkaline, aqueous solution of glutaraldehyde buffered with a sodium phenate system to a pH of 7.4 to form a complex of glutaraldehyde and phenate. When used for high-level disinfection, one part of the activated solution is diluted with 15 parts of tap water (1:16 dilution).

Actions and uses
Glutaraldehyde phenate solution is activated before use by mixing a phenate buffer with glutaraldehyde. It remains active for 30 days. The undiluted solution is used for sterilisation of instruments and is sporicidal against aerobic and anaerobic spores.

When diluted (1:16) for high-level disinfection, glutaraldehyde phenate will destroy vegetative bacteria, and hydrophilic and lipophilic viruses in the tubercle bacillus in 10 minutes. Directions should be followed and all items pre-cleaned before immersion.

Adverse reactions and precautions
Glutaraldehyde phenate solution can cause irritation of the skin, eyes, and mucous membrane. Contact should be avoided by using eye protection, utility gloves, and a mask.

Chlorine preparations

Sodium hypochlorite solutions

Sodium hypochlorite is available as household bleach. A solution of 1 part of 5% sodium hypochlorite with 9 parts of water (1:10 dilution) will provide a disinfectant solution containing 0.5% or 5,000 ppm sodium hypochlorite. The diluted solution is prepared fresh daily, because it is not stable and will degrade upon exposure to air.

If sodium hypochlorite is used as a disinfectant, preclean the surfaces, as excess organic material will react with the available chlorine and reduce the disinfectant efficiency. A 10-minute contact time is necessary. It is usually used as a surface disinfectant, and also as an immersion disinfectant in prosthodontics.

Adverse reactions and precautions
Sodium hypochlorite solution may irritate skin, eyes, and mucous membranes.

Do not mix with other household chemicals such as toilet-bowl cleaners, rust removers, and products containing acid or ammonia.

It is corrosive to metals, especially aluminium, and solutions discolour fabric or clothing.

Chlorous acid and chlorine dioxide

Chlorous acid and chlorine dioxide are generated by the combination of sodium chlorite and an organic acid. The products available at present in this category provide high-level disinfection in 3 minutes. They may be sprayed or wiped onto surfaces to be disinfected.

Adverse reactions and precautions
Prolonged, repeated exposure will result in surface oxidation of certain metals.

There have been reports of mucous membrane sensitivity. Care should be taken to keep the stored solution in closed containers. If coughing, wheezing, or difficulty in breathing are caused by its use on large surface areas or in confined spaces, move to fresh air at once and avoid reuse.

Phenols

These chemicals are not recommended by the EPA for either immersion or surface disinfection. Phenols are highly effective against certain micro-organisms, however some can withstand their action.

Combination synthetic phenolics

Combination synthetic phenolics currently accepted for disinfecting purposes in dentistry contain *o*-phenylphenol 9% and *o*-benzyl-*p*-chlorophenol 1%.

Actions and uses

When used at room temperature, these products may be diluted 1:32 for disinfection.

Combination phenolics are bactericidal, tuberculocidal, fungicidal, and virucidal, but have not been shown to be sporicidal at room temperature.

These compounds may be used as surface and immersion disinfectants. Disinfection requires a 10-minute contact time. These solutions should be mixed fresh daily. They do not have negative handling characteristics or objectionable odours, but may damage plastic and rubber.

Iodophors

An iodophor is a weak complex of elemental iodine or triiodide, with a carrier that serves to increase the solubility of the iodine, and provides a slow iodine release. These solutions usually contain soap additives, which is useful when pre-cleaning surfaces.

Actions and uses

Iodophor disinfectants are diluted for use, according to the directions on the product label. In most cases this is a dilution of 1:213, i.e. 1 part of disinfectant solution to 212 parts of water; this dilution provides an optimal amount of free iodine. These compounds are more active in aqueous solution than in alcohol.

Iodophors are used as surface or immersion disinfectants, and are effective against a wide variety of micro-organisms including *Mycobacterium tuberculosis*. They are not approved as sterilants.

For use on surfaces, the solution may be sprayed on using a spray bottle to wet the surface completely. The product should remain on the surface for 10 minutes, or for the time recommended on the product label. Prepare fresh solutions daily.

These compounds may stain some materials, particularly vinyl upholstery, and it is advisable to test the iodophor on a small test area before extensive use on environmental surfaces. Cleaning the surfaces periodically with soap and water or an iodophor neutraliser (e.g. Promedyne, Cottrell Ltd) may reduce this discoloration.

Adverse reactions and precautions

Iodophors are usually safe, non-irritant disinfectants, but some cases of skin staining and irritation have been reported. It is advisable to wear utility gloves, eye protection, and a mask when mixing and using these solutions.

Quaternary ammonium compounds

The quaternary ammonium compounds are not accepted by the EPA for use in dentistry because of their limited antimicrobial activity. Examples of such compounds are, benzalkonium chloride and dibenzalkoniumchloride.

Alcohols

The EPA and ADA do not recommend the use of alcohols in dentistry, either as surface or as immersion disinfectants.

Alcohols may be combined with a low concentration of synthetic phenolics; this action can be synergistic. These solutions may be used for surface disinfection of pre-cleaned surfaces. (See Chapter 7.)

Peroxygenated compounds

These are recently introduced disinfectants which release nascent oxygen and contain a detergent. They are user-friendly and may be of use for surface disinfection. They are not at present recommended by the EPA.

Summary of disinfectants

Table 8.1 summarises those types and brands of disinfectants used in dentistry which are recommended by the ADA. Such disinfectants must be registered with the EPA as a hospital disinfectant and must be tuberculocidal. Virucidal activity must include as a minimum both lipophilic and hydrophilic viruses.

Table 8.1   Types and brands of disinfectants recommended by ADA.

Chemical	Usual application	Chemical	Usual application

Chlorine compounds
  Alcide
  Exspore
  Bleach
	Surface disinfection	2% Glutaraldehyde neutral
		  Glutarex
			Sterilant and high-level immersion disinfectant

Iodophors
  Biocide
  Surf-A-cide
  Pro-Medyn-D
	Surface disinfection	2% Glutaraldeyde acidic
		  Banicide
		  Sterall
		  Wavicide 01
			Sterilant and high-level immersion disinfectant

Combination synthetic
    phenolics
  Dentaseptic
  Multicide
  Omni II
	Surface disinfection or immersion disinfectant	2% Glutaraldehyde alkaline
		    activated
		  Cidex 7
		  Glutall
		  Omnicide
		  Procide 14
			Sterilant and high-level immersion disinfectant

2% Glutaraldeyde with
    phenolic buffer
  Sporacidin
	Sterilant & high-level immersion disinfectant		

A *full* list of currently accepted products may be obtained by contacting the Office of the Council on Dental Therapeutics ADA.

Other disinfectants available are summarised in **Table 8.2.** These are not approved by the EPA and ADA.

Table 8.2   Available disinfectants not approved by ADA & EPA.

Chemical	Application

Alcohol plus additives
    Microzid, Hibispray
    Lysol
    Citrace
	Surface disinfection

Peroxygenated
    compounds
    Virkon
	Surface disinfection

Sterilisation using Chemical Solutions

Thoroughly clean the items to be sterilised. Read the product label, checking that the chemical is sporocidal. A 2% w/v alkaline glutaraldehyde is recommended.

Put the clean, dry items into the chemical, covering them completely. Leave them immersed for the time recommended on the product label (this can be as long as 10 hours). Remove items from the chemical solution with a sterile instrument and rinse them with sterile water. Dry with sterile towels and store under sterile conditions.

This method of sterilisation is usually impractical in dental practice. However it is of use occasionally to sterilise semi-critical items, which are damaged by heat.

Sterilisation using liquid chemicals has the following major disadvantages:

- The solutions must be changed regularly; this is expensive.
- The effectiveness cannot be checked.
- Toxic fumes require special ventilation.
- It cannot be used with packaged items.
- The long immersion times are unrealistic in a busy practice.
- The method rusts and damages certain instruments.

High-Level Disinfection

Immersion in chemical solutions for shorter periods will achieve high-level disinfection, i.e. the destruction, of vegetative forms of micro-organisms but *not* of spores.

- Read the label to see that the chemical kills spores – 2% w/v alkaline glutaraldehyde is recommended.
- Place the clean, dry items into the chemical, covering them completely. Leave them immersed for the *shorter* time shown on the product label.
- Remove the items and rinse thoroughly with water to remove all chemical residue.
- Dry with disposable towels.
- Use items immediately or store in a sterilised container.

Precautions

If a chemical is moved from its original container, the new container must be labelled. Tanks containing disinfectants should be covered to prevent oxidation or the release of irritant vapours.

Accidental exposure to chemicals

The Poison Control telephone number must be displayed in a convenient position. Antidotes should be available for use after accidental exposure.

If solutions contact the skin or mucous membrane, wash thoroughly with water.

Eyewash Stations

Eyewash solutions must be kept in an eyewash station located in a convenient position.

If eyes are exposed to a chemical, flood them with plain water (**8.2**).

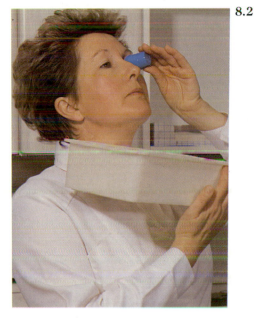

8.2

8.2 Flood the eyes with plain water, if exposed to chemicals.

OSHA regulations

Various eyewash systems, ranging from inexpensive eyewash bottles or faucet attachments, to elaborate separately plumbed systems, are available from laboratory or safety companies.

The current Occupational Safety and Health Administration (OSHA) regulations state:

'Where the eyes or body of any person may be exposed to corrosive materials, suitable facilities for quick drenching or flushing of the eyes and body shall be provided within the work area for immediate emergency use.'

The ambiguity of the current regulation means that each employer must use his/her own judgement about how best to satisfy the eyewash requirement. For further advice, contact the ADA.

References

[1]Overton, D., Burgess, J., Beck, B., Matis, B. Glutaraldehyde test kits. Evaluation for accuracy and range. *General Dent.*, 1989;**37**:126–8.

[2]Klier, D., Tucker, J., Averbach, R. Clinical evaluation of glutaraldehyde non-biological monitors. *Quintessence Int.*, 1989;**20**:271–7.

[3]Hess, J., Molinari, J., Gleason, M., Radecki, C. Epidermal toxicity of disinfectants. *Am. J. Dent.*, 1991;**4**:51–6.

9. Instrument Arrangement and Packaging

Instruments, cotton goods, and other disposable materials used for specific dental procedures are arranged in appropriate trays, packages, or sterilisation pouches. Careful organisation of these helps the dental team to implement procedures efficiently and facilitates a well-organised cross infection control programme.

If possible, wrap or package everything that must be kept sterile and that will not be used immediately.

Dental Trays

Covered metal trays

The standard-size aluminium dental tray (**9.1**) is very popular in the UK. The base of the tray is perforated to facilitate free movement of steam or chemical vapour. A paper tray liner is used to cover the tray-base perforations; this minimises external contamination during the brief storage period.

Sets of instruments which are reused *quickly*, e.g. instruments for routine restorative procedures, may be sterilised on open trays. After completion of the sterilisation cycle, a disinfected solid lid is placed over the tray (**9.2**).

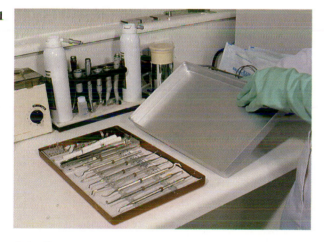

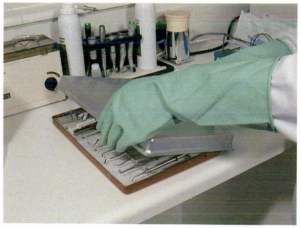

9.1   Instruments contained in a standard metal tray, a solid, well fitting lid is used, with a paper tray liner.

9.2   Placing a solid lid over the tray is suitable for a short storage period.

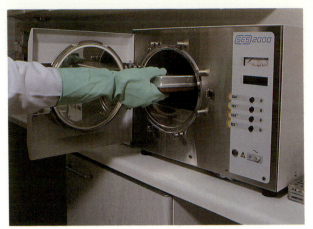

Some autoclaves have shelves which are wide enough to allow sterilisation of both trays and lids (**9.3**). If a solid lid is used in an autoclave, it is left slightly open to allow steam to enter. After completion of the autoclave cycle, the lid is tightly closed.

Trays which are to be stored for longer periods, may be covered with a tight-fitting, perforated lid, wrapped in steam-permeable paper, which is sealed with autoclave tape (**9.4**).

Small trays, suitable for examination kits, are available (**9.5**).

9.3 Trays and lids may be sterilised together in some autoclaves.

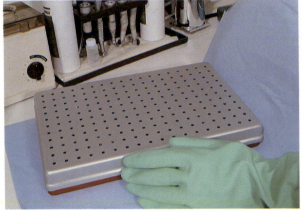

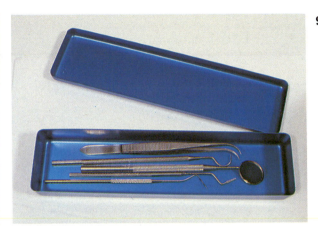

9.4 Trays stored for longer periods have perforated lids and are wrapped in paper.

9.5 A tray which is useful for examinations.

Practical recommendations

- Store trays away from aerosol and dust, on shelves which are disinfected weekly (**9.6**).
- Stack trays in such a way that the tray stored the longest is taken out for use first.
- Never overload a tray; free circulation of steam is essential.
- Arrange instruments, cotton goods, and dis-

posables in the same procedural order on each tray. This is not only efficient, but helps avoid the chance of an accidental injury from a misplaced contaminated sharp instrument.

- Place a chemical time/temperature indicator strip into each lidded tray before sterilisation (**9.7**).

9.6

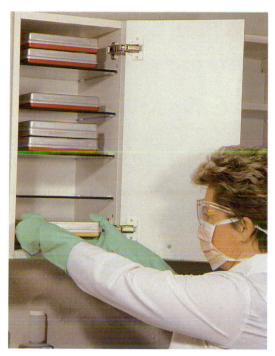

9.6 Trays stored away from dirty areas.

9.7

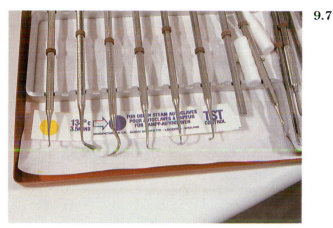

9.7 A TST strip is placed in a tray before autoclaving.

IMS instrument cassettes

IMS cassettes are becoming popular in the USA. They are lightweight resin cassettes which have a 12–18 instrument capacity and a section designed to hold disposables and miscellaneous items (**9.8**).

The open design of the IMS cassette enables instruments to be cleaned *within* the cassette and eliminates potentially dangerous handling of contaminated instruments during the cleaning and distribution process.

9.8

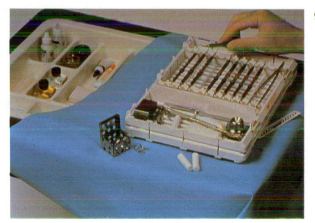

9.8 The IMS cassette. (Courtesy Hu Friedy.)

Using the IMS cassette

After completion of the dental procedure, place the instruments back on the cassette in the correct procedural order. Close the cassette and clean, using either an ultrasonic cleaner for 12 minutes followed by thorough rinsing[1] (**9.9**), or a dishwasher-type cleaner.

Place an IMS indicator strip inside the cassette, together with cotton wool materials and other disposables.

Wrap the cassette in IMS autoclave wrap (**9.10**) and seal this with IMS monitor tape which indicates that the cassette has passed through the sterilisation cycle and also identifies the contents.

After sterilisation, store the cassettes in aseptic conditions until their next use (**9.11**). Do not use if the wrap is torn or unsealed.

Certain chemicals and detergents can cause discoloration and/or corrosion of cassettes. Further information is provided in the operator's manual. A steriliser and ultrasonic cleaner compatibility list is provided by the manufacturer.

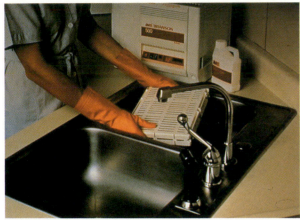

9.9 Rinsing after ultrasonic cleaning. (Courtesy Hu Friedy.)

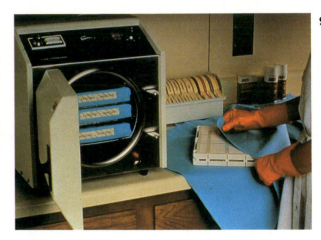

9.10 Wrapping the IMS cassette. (Courtesy Hu Friedy.)

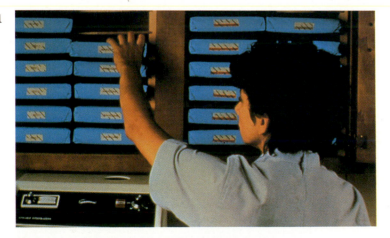

9.11 Storing IMS cassettes. (Courtesy Hu Friedy.)

General recommendations

Wherever possible use trays rather than sterilisation pouches and wraps. The advantages of trays are that they:

- Allow instruments to be set up in an organised way.
- Restrict gross contamination to a surface which

can be cleaned and sterilised.
- Provide safe, aseptic storage (pouches and paper wraps may be penetrated by sharp instruments).

Trays are particularly useful for sets of larger instruments.

Sterilisation Pouches

Pouches are very useful for the sterilisation and aseptic storage of single instruments, or small sets of instruments which are infrequently used, e.g. forceps and elevators.

In the UK, the Department of Health (DOH) has issued a warning (FPN 497) to all dentists about sterilisers which rely on the displacement of air by

steam alone. These should not be used to sterilise instruments contained in sterilisation pouches.

However, studies have shown that instruments within pouches can be sterilised in non-vacuum autoclaves.[2] Each pouch should be flatted by hand, to drive out most of the air, and must contain a chemical time/temperature indicator strip.

Clearview sterilisation pouches

Clearview sterilisation pouches enable easy identification of the contents of the pouch and the colour change of a chemical indicator can be observed without opening the pouch (**9.12**). Self-seal clearview pouches are available.

Items within sterile dental pouches (single-wall

paper, sealed nylon, and paper/plastic pouches) may be safely stored for one year.[3] It is advisable to dry pouches before they are stored for long periods. Certain autoclaves incorporate pouch racks which facilitate quick drying (**9.13**).

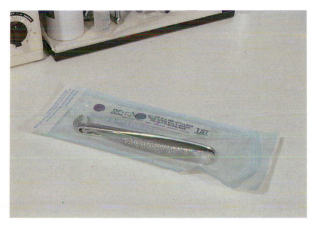

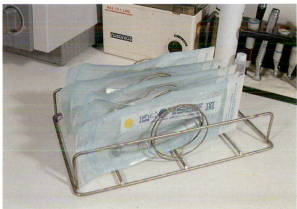

9.13

9.12   A clearview sterilisation pouch, containing forceps and a TST strip.

9.13   The SES 2000 pouch rack.

Other types of pouches and packaging

All-paper, self-seal sterilisation pouches are available. The contents of these cannot be easily identified, except by a written record on the pouch. Ink should not be used to mark pouches—use a soft lead pencil.

Muslin may be used as a wrap and sealed with the appropriate tape. Nylon bags can be used for dental surgical instruments, if the bags are heat-sealed or taped, rather than stapled. A reliable brand of nylon bag which is manufactured to a precise thickness should be used.

Pouches, packaging, and sharp instruments

Sharp points of instruments may pierce paper, plastic, or muslin and this compromises aseptic storage. Gauze or heavy paper wrapped around the sharp tips will help to prevent this.

Note: In the USA longer time cycles are used for wrapped materials (see Chapter 10).

References

[1]Miller, C. and Hardwick, L. Ultrasonic cleaning of dental instruments in cassettes. *General Dent.*, 1988;**36**:31–6.
[2]Wood, P. R. and Martin, M. V. A study of autoclave bags in non-vacuum autoclaves. *J. Dent.*, 1989;**17**:148–9.
[3]Schwartz, R. and Davis, R. Safe storage times for sterilisation pouches. *Oral. Surg.*, 1990;**3**:297–300.

10. Sterilisation of Instruments

Critical and semi-critical items and instruments are sterilised, if possible, by heat.

Sterilisation is the process by which all forms of micro-organisms are destroyed, including bacteria, viruses, fungi, and spores.

There are four distinct stages which achieve safe instrument sterilisation:

- Pre-cleaning disinfection, using 'holding' solutions.
- Pre-sterilisation cleaning.
- Sterilisation.
- Aseptic storage.

The Sterilisation Area

The area for cleaning and sterilisation needs careful planning, with a generous amount of room allowed for wide worktops, a sink, an ultrasonic cleaner, and steriliser(s).

Some offices have a separate central sterilisation area. This should be easily accessible to all the separate surgeries in the practice. Instruments must be carried safely to surgery areas; closed trays, baskets, or trolleys are recommended.

Many offices locate the sterilisation area within the surgery. If this is the case, it should be situated away from the operating area. The layout of the sterilisation area is illustrated (**10.1, 10.2**).

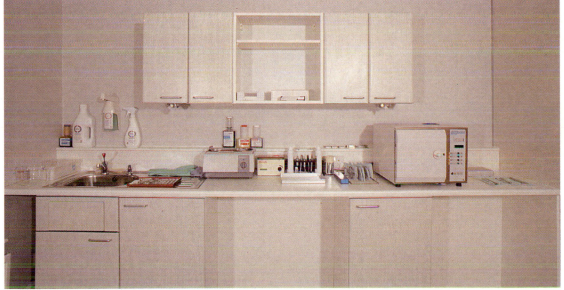

10.1

10.1   The sterilisation area.

Dirty area	Sink	Cleaning area	Ultrasonic bath	Packaging area	Steriliser	Clean area
Area of high contamination				**Area of medium contamination**	**Area of low contamination**	

10.2

10.2   Layout of the sterilisation area.

Dirty area

Trays containing contaminated instruments and disposables are taken to this area after use. Disposables are placed carefully in a waste receiver.

Sink

A deep sink with elbow- or foot-operated tap controls and an efficient splashback is essential. A deep sink is necessary to minimise splashing when washing or rinsing instruments.

This sink is for cleaning only. A separate sink, located nearby, should be reserved for hand washing. Decontamination of rubber utility gloves may be carried out in the cleaning sink. Instruments in holding baths are rinsed and then taken to the cleaning area.

Cleaning area

After removal of contaminated disposable items, instruments and trays are taken to the cleaning area, where they are organised into baskets prior to ultrasonic cleaning.

If trays cannot be ultrasonically cleaned, they are wiped clean in this area, which should be sufficiently large for several trays.

Ultrasonic bath

Choose a good-quality product which cleans large numbers of widely spaced instruments. (*See* section on ultrasonic cleaning, p.116.)

If the cleaner is located in a surgery, the noise when it is in use may be distracting. Consider this when purchasing an ultrasonic cleaner.

A low-volume continuous air evacuation system is located near to the cleaning and ultrasonic bath area, and the vapours vented *outside* the room.

Packaging area

After cleaning, instruments are thoroughly rinsed and taken to the packaging area where they are dried and then either loaded into trays, placed in pouches, or wrapped. Trays are wrapped in this area.

Sterilisation pouches, paper wraps, chemical indicator strips, etc., are stored in cupboards above the packaging area.

Steriliser

A good-quality autoclave capable of holding standard trays or IMS cassettes is essential. Ideally, a second steriliser, such as a chemiclave, is located in this area for use both as a back-up and to sterilise instruments which would be damaged by autoclaving.

Clean area

Hot trays and packaged instruments are taken from the steriliser to this area before being stored in adjacent closed cabinets.

Precautions

Adequate lighting is essential to facilitate careful inspection and handling of instruments.

Heavy rubber utility gloves, protective eyewear, a mask, and a plastic apron should be worn when performing the decontamination stages of sterilisation.

Pre-Sterilisation Disinfection

After use, place instruments into a disinfectant detergent solution in a container located within the operating zone near to the dentist (**10.3**).

At the end of the dental procedure, take the container to the sterilisation area. Thoroughly rinse the instruments with water (**10.4**). The solution is reused but should be discarded daily.

Place heavily contaminated endodontic files and rotary instruments into a small volume of holding solution contained in a beaker located on the bracket table tray (**10.5**). Discard holding solution, rinse the instruments, and add ultrasonic solution to the beaker, then suspend this in an ultrasonic bath.

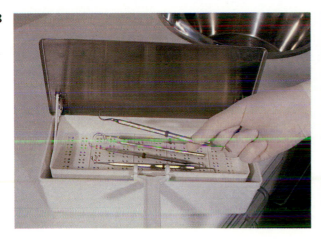

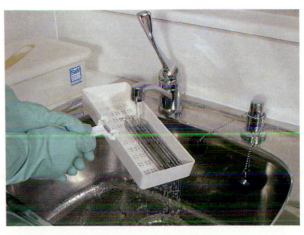

10.3 Container of holding solution near to the dentist.

10.4 Rinsing instruments after immersion in holding solution. This type of container facilitates easy rinsing of instruments.

Holding instruments in disinfectant solutions shortly after use has two benefits:

- There is minimal drying of blood, pus, and saliva on instruments, which makes them easier to clean.
- Instruments are safer to handle during the subsequent sterilisation stages because of the disinfectant action of the holding solution.

A synthetic phenolic solution, diluted 1:32, is an ideal holding solution.

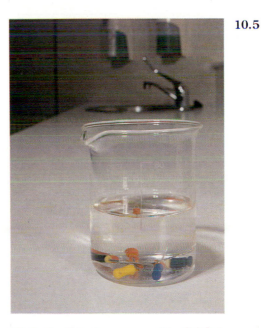

10.5 Small beakers are used to disinfect rotary and endodontic instruments.

Pre-Sterilisation Cleaning

Proteinaceous material protects micro-organisms on the surface of instruments from heat and other sterilisation conditions. Pre-sterilisation cleaning may be achieved in one of three ways:

- Hand scrubbing
- Ultrasonic cleaning
- Dishwasher instrument cleaning.

Heavy rubber utility gloves, protective eyewear, a mask, and a plastic apron should be worn when decontaminating instruments in the sterilisation area.

Hand scrubbing of instruments

10.6

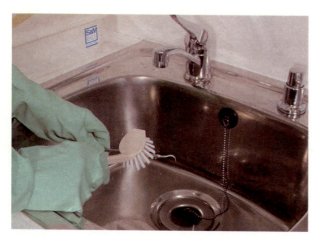

10.6 Long-handled brush.

Hand scrubbing increases the chance of injury from contaminated instruments and from contact with contaminated fluids. This method of cleaning should be avoided if at all possible.

If an item must be manually scrubbed, splatter should be kept to a minimum. This is achieved by scrubbing under water in a deep sink, *not* under fast-running water from a tap. A long-handled brush is always used (**10.6**).

Ultrasonic cleaning

Several studies have shown that, when performed correctly, ultrasonic cleaning will remove dried serum,[1] whole blood,[2] plaque,[3] zinc phosphate cement,[2,4] and polycarboxylate cement[2] from instruments, metal surfaces, and dentures. It has been found to be more effective than manual cleaning.[5]

Ultrasonic cleaning minimises the handling of contaminated instruments by the nurse and reduces the chance of injuries from sharp, contaminated instruments.

Instruments are loaded into a *metal* basket which is then placed into the ultrasonic bath (**10.7**). The unit is activated for the time recommended by the manufacturer (usually about 6 minutes). Instruments which are contained in cassettes are cleaned for 12 minutes.[6]

After the cleaning cycle is complete, the basket is taken to the sink and the instruments are carefully and thoroughly rinsed under tap water (**10.8**). The instruments are checked for residual debris which may be safely removed manually.

Instruments are taken to the packaging area, where they are unloaded from the baskets onto a thick disposable paper towel. The instruments are thoroughly 'pat' dried using strong paper towels. *Drying is important* (**10.9**).

Small rotary and endodontic instruments should be held in beakers of ultrasonic cleaning solution which are suspended in the cleaning bath (**10.10**).

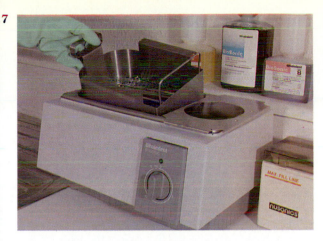

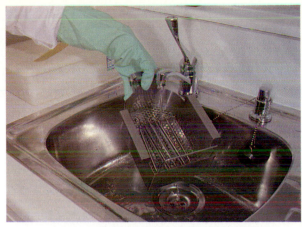

10.7 Baskets of instruments loaded into an ultrasonic bath.

10.8 Rinse away all traces of ultrasonic solution.

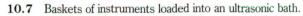
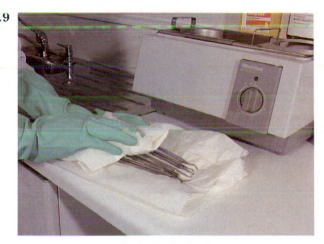

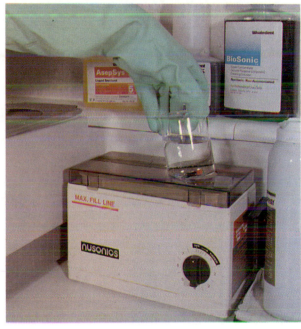

10.9 Drying after ultrasonic cleaning is essential.

10.10 Beakers used for small instruments.

Precautions

- Activate a new solution by operating the unit for 2 minutes, without instruments in the reservoir.
- Instruments should be totally submerged in the ultrasonic solution. Keep the reservoir a half to three-quarters full of solution.
- Do not overfill baskets with instruments, and do not place loose instruments at the bottom of the tank. This decreases cleaning effectiveness.
- Place a tight-fitting lid on the unit during cleaning.
- Use a basket with handles, to minimise hand contact with the ultrasonic solution.
- Use an ultrasonic solution that is recommended by the manufacturer. Some ultrasonic solutions contain disinfectants which enhance the decontamination cycle.[7] Avoid acidic ultrasonic solutions which damage instruments.[8]
- The ultrasonic solution should be changed at least *once* a day. At the end of the day, clean, disinfect, rinse, and dry the chamber and leave it empty overnight.
- Check the cleaner periodically by placing a 102 × 102 mm piece of regular aluminium foil (Reynolds wrap, regular weight, about 16 μm thickness) into an activated solution (**10.11**). After 5 minutes, small holes should appear in the foil if the cleaner is working efficiently.
- To achieve optimum results, follow the manufacturer's instructions for use and care.

10.11

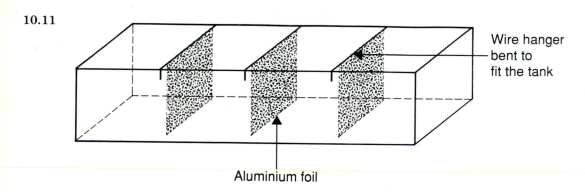

Wire hanger bent to fit the tank

Aluminium foil

10.11   To test the efficiency of the ultrasonic cleaner: the aluminium foil should not touch the bottom or the sides of the reservoir.

Ultrasonic cleaners and solutions

The following ultrasonic cleaners were recommended by the Clinical Research Associates (CRA):[9]

BIOSONIC — Whaledent
T33C — Health Sonics Group

COLSTER 3 — Provides ultrasonic clean, rinse, and dry, but is noisy.

Details of these cleaners are given in the report.

Dishwasher instrument cleaners

These machines are popular in Germany and Scandinavia. Dishwasher cleaners are capable of holding either instrument sets in cassettes or single instruments in containers (**10.12**).

The machines first pre-rinse the instruments at a low temperature, to prevent the coagulation of proteins. Washing then takes place at 90°C for 10 minutes using recommended disinfectant/detergent and instruments are dry after the cycle is completed.

Larger models (**10.13**) are available for use in central sterilisation rooms.

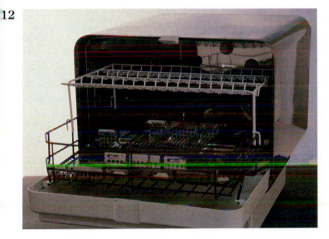

10.12   A cleaner suitable for use in a single surgery. (Courtesy Eschman Ltd.)

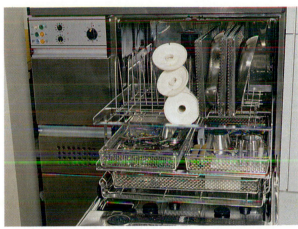

10.13   A cleaner suitable for use in central sterilisation rooms. (Courtesy Prof. Hurlen, Oslo University.)

Sterilisation

Instruments must be clean *and* dry before sterilisation.

There are four types of sterilisers used routinely in dentistry:

- The steam autoclave.
- The chemical vapour pressure steriliser.
- The dry heat oven.
- The glass bead/salt steriliser.

Sterilisers sold in the USA are regulated by two agencies. The Food and Drug Administration (FDA) is responsible for devices of all kinds, while the Environmental Protection Agency (EPA) limits its responsibility to procedures involving the discharge of harmful chemicals.

The steam autoclave

A steam autoclave sterilises by the use of steam under pressure.

Non-vacuum autoclaves are used in dental practice. These use incoming steam pressure to evacuate air. Many good quality, modern, non-vacuum autoclaves are very efficient in air removal if the autoclave is not overloaded.

A prescribed temperature, pressure, and time are necessary to destroy bacterial spores. The temperature–time combinations for autoclaves are shown in **Tables 10.1** and **10.2**. The faster, higher temperature cycles are generally favoured by dentists in general practice.

Autoclaves in the USA have a wider range of cycles available (**10.14**) than those in the UK, and American authorities advise that wrapped instrument loads can be sterilised using a portable steam autoclave.

Table 10.1 Temperature and time combinations recommended for autoclaves in the UK.

Temperature °C (pressure)	Minimum hold time
134–138 (207 kPa; 30 lb/in^2)	3 min
121–124 (103.5 kPa; 15 lb/in^2)	15 min

Table 10.2 Temperature and time combinations recommended for autoclaves in the USA.

	Temperature °C (pressure)	Minimum hold time
Unwrapped items	132 (270 kPa; 30 lb/in^2)	3 min
	121 (103.5 kPa; 15 lb/in^2)	15 min
Lightly wrapped items	132 (270 kPa; 30 lb/in^2)	8 min
	121 (103.5 kPa; 15 lb/in^2)	20 min
Heavily wrapped items	132 (270 kPa; 30 lb/in^2)	10 min
	121 (103.5 kPa; 15 lb/in^2)	20 min

10.14

10.14 Additional cycles are available for sterilising wrapped loads.

Purchasing an autoclave

The majority of new models are fully automatic. Choose a good quality product with good service back-up. Compare the features of an autoclave with those described in the UK or USA evaluation programmes.

Evaluation programmes

USA
The Council on Dental Materials, Instruments and Equipment has an acceptance programme for steam autoclaves. Steam autoclave sterilisers are required to:

- Be listed by Underwriter's Laboratory.
- Meet the American Society of Mechanical Engineers boiler and pressure vessel code requirements.

- Reach and maintain 121°C at 103.5 kPa (15 lb/in^2) for 45 minutes and 132°C at 186.3 kPa (27 lb/in^2) for 15 minutes.
- Have the means to remove air, measure steam temperature and pressure, and check operation.
- Have an instruction manual.
- Have been evaluated for ability to sterilise, i.e. destroy bacterial spores.

Two other points that need to be considered are:

Drying cycle: some steam autoclaves have a 'drying cycle'. Dry instruments in trays and packages may be stored safely for long periods without corrosion.

Chamber size: the chamber size of an autoclave should be large enough to allow the sterilisation of standard trays or IMS cassettes.

Directions for use

Use the cycles listed in **Tables 10.1** (UK) and **10.2** (USA). These should not be interrupted. Minimise trapped air in the autoclave chamber, taking the following precautions:

- Do *not* overload the trays (**10.15**).
- Load the trays carefully, to allow free circulation of steam round the instruments (**10.16**).
- Use trays with perforated bases to allow air displacement and free steam circulation.
- If lidded trays are to be sterilised, fit perforated lids. Take solid lids off trays before sterilisation.
- Separate packaged or wrapped items, do not stack together.
- Do not overload the autoclave with trays and pouches.
- Sterilisation failure in a steam autoclave can usually be avoided if proper cleansing, packaging, and loading precautions are observed.
- Remove all particles of amalgam, cements, or other filling materials, which adhere to instruments, after ultrasonic cleaning. This will avoid clogging up the chamber and prevent impaired operation of the solenoid and the air-vent valve.
- Rinse disinfectants and cleansers from instruments. Contaminated water in the reservoir will cause the air-vent valve to fail, and will increase the likelihood of instrument corrosion.
- Some manufacturers recommend using distilled or deionised water in autoclaves. In 'hard water' areas, tap water will form scaled deposits in the water chamber. Chemicals in the water may also affect the operation of the valve and the filter.

UK

Portable steam sterilisers should meet BS 3970 part 1 and part 4 1990. The Department of Health (DOH) tested a number of small steam sterilisers; the results were summarised in a report[10] which was issued to all practitioners. The test summaries should be considered only in conjunction with the full test reports,[11,12] before a decision to purchase is made.

The dangers of autoclaves, and advice on their use, are the subjects of a guidance note from the Health and Safety Executive (HSE).[13]

The DOH does not recommend portable autoclaves, of the type used in dental practice, for the sterilisation of wrapped instruments or instruments in pouches. Studies, however, have indicated that it is possible to sterilise instruments in pouches at 134°C for 3 minutes.[14]

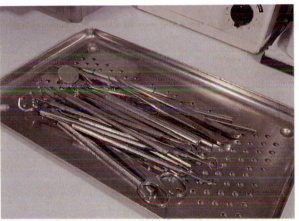

10.15

10.15 Autoclave tray overloaded with instruments.

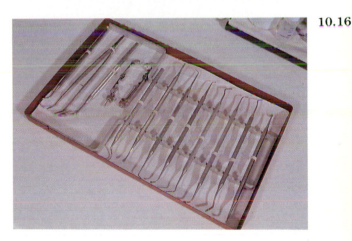

10.16

10.16 Correct loading of sterilisation tray.

Items suitable for autoclaving

The steam autoclave is suitable for the sterilisation of:

- High-quality stainless steel instruments.
- Handpieces which can be autoclaved.
- Cloth goods.

- Glass slabs, dishes, stones. Stones should be *dry*, wet stones may rupture under steam sterilisation.
- Large, plastic suction tips.
- Packaged and wrapped instruments (*see* Chapter 9).
- Heat-resistant, plastic instruments.

Limitations of use

Carbon-steel instruments will rust after a limited number of autoclave cycles. It is sometimes recommended that, prior to autoclaving, instruments which are susceptible to rust should be treated with a non-toxic, non-silicone, oil emulsion. This tends to reduce rust and lubricates instruments without leaving a noticeable oily or sticky film. These emulsions do not impair sterilisation. Commercial chemicals and 2% w/v sodium nitrite are used to reduce rusting and corrosion.[15,16]

Needles should not be autoclaved, nor oil, wax, and dry powder.

Autoclave maintenance

Simple maintenance can be carried out by surgery staff:

- Clean the chamber *weekly* with a weak detergent and rinse well (**10.17**).
- Clean the gasket weekly, applying a recommended silicone compound to it.

- Check the level of the reservoir *twice daily*. Do not overfill the reservoir or fill during the cycle, since this may cause flooding at the end of the cycle.
- Empty the water reservoir *weekly* and remove particles on the chamber floor using high-velocity aspiration (**10.18**). Flush the chamber through with 2 litres of water.

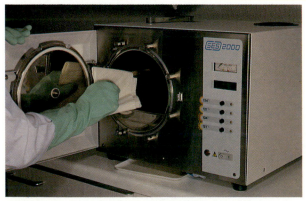

10.17 Cleaning the autoclave chamber.

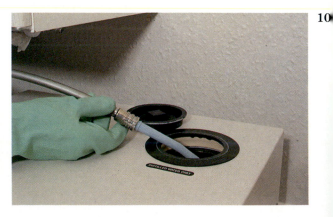

10.18 Cleaning the water reservoir of the autoclave.

Servicing

All pressure vessels, including autoclaves, must be regularly maintained. Autoclaves can be an explosive risk if the door is not secured, or they are not maintained properly.

Autoclaves should be inspected and certified for insurance purposes annually. In the UK, the Dentist Provident Society can arrange regular autoclave ex-aminations through Ajax Engineering Policies at Lloyds; safety certificates are issued and these should be retained.

An autoclave should be regularly checked and should be serviced at intervals recommended by the manufacturers. *This is important.*

The Statim cassette autoclave

The Statim autoclave (**10.19**) is a compact table-top autoclave, designed for rapid sterilisation of instruments. The autoclave has a drying cycle. Instruments are sterilised in closed cassettes into which steam is introduced after air has been removed. A 6-minute cycle is available for unwrapped instruments, and a 12-minute cycle for wrapped instruments.

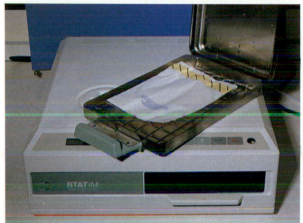

10.19

10.19   The Statim autoclave. (Courtesy Dr M.V. Martin.)

Chemical vapour sterilisers

Chemical vapour sterilisers operate by heating a deodorised alcohol, formaldehyde, and ethylmethyl ketone solution, which can be obtained from the manufacturer, to 132°C at 138–276 kPa (20–40 lb/in^2) for 20 minutes in a closed chamber.

The chemical vapour steriliser offers three main advantages:

- A fairly short cycle—a total of 30 minutes. Short 'flash cycles' of 7 minutes are now available on new models, when sterilising unwrapped items.
- Instruments do not dull, rust, or corrode; this extends their useful life.
- Instruments are dry at the end of the cycle.

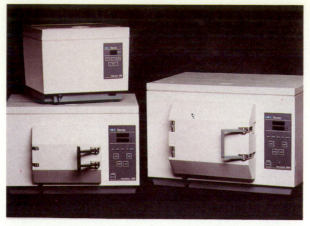

10.20 The Chemiclave models 7000 and 8000, with the ultrasonic cleaner.

The main disadvantages are that good ventilation is essential to eliminate residual formaldehyde vapours from the chamber, and the extra cost of purchasing sterilising solutions, e.g. vaposteril solution used in the chemiclave.

In newer models, such as the Chemiclave 7000 and 8000 (**10.20**), the volume of residual vapour is minimised. If the chemiclave is operated in a poorly ventilated area, a **chemipurge** system should be used which absorbs the vapours.

Note: The formaldehyde exposure limit permitted by OSHA is 1 ppm as an 8-hour, time-weighted average and the 15-min short exposure is 2 ppm.[17] If the unit is operated in accordance with instructions, the levels of formaldehyde emitted are *below* the levels allowed under the new OSHA standards.

Directions for use

- Instruments must be clean and dry before sterilising in a chemiclave. Wet instruments could increase the water content of the vapour above the 15% threshold level at which rusting and corrosion of instruments is possible.
- Use recommended pouches, which allow penetration of the alcohol–formaldehyde vapour.
- Do not wrap instruments in heavy paper, muslin, or nylon.
- If trays are used, they must be perforated and uncovered.

Instruments suitable for sterilisation with chemical vapour

The chemical vapour steriliser is suitable for:

All dental hand instruments.
Handpieces—the majority of good-quality handpieces can be sterilised using the Chemiclave 7000 or 8000 but the manufacturer's recommendations should be followed.
Carbon-steel and diamond burs.
Endodontic instruments.
Orthodontic wires and bands.
Orthodontic pliers, where rusting of the joints may cause problems.

Maintenance and servicing

It is *essential* that the manufacturer's maintenance and servicing recommendations are carefully followed. Clean the chamber weekly with MDT chamber cleaner and special pads (Scotchbrite by 3M or MDT pads).

Dry-heat sterilisers

Dry heat is an effective means of sterilisation, when it is used *properly*.

Unwrapped, moderate loads of instruments placed in an oven can be sterilised at 160–170°C in 1 hour. Wrapped loads require a longer time exposure.

The standard dry-heat oven (**10.21**), which is manufactured for dental use, is *not* recommended for a busy dental practice for the following reasons:

- Low-temperature pockets in the chamber during a sterilisation cycle may prevent sterilisation of the load.[18] Circulation fans which are fitted to more sophisticated ovens may not overcome this problem.[18]
- The complete cycle, i.e. warming-up time, sterilisation time, and cooling-down time, is very long (approximately 90 minutes) and unsuitable in a busy dental practice.
- Most ovens *do not* have a door-locking system, which allows interruption of the sterilisation cycle. If cycles are interrupted, loads are not sterile.
- Turbine handpieces are damaged if heated to a temperature of 160°C.
- Loads of wrapped or enclosed instruments are sterilised using dry heat, however the time to achieve sterilisation at 160°C is unpredictable. This supports the suggestion that dry heat sterilisation must be tested under actual conditions for

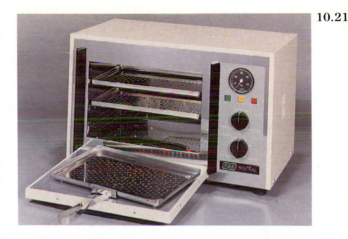

10.21

10.21   The dry-heat oven.

use, and be monitored with spore strips.[19]

- There is no certification or acceptance programme for dry heat sterilisers in the USA.[19] In the UK, British Standard 3421:1961 is a specification for performance of electrically heated sterilising ovens.

Rapid dry-heat sterilisation

The Cox rapid dry-heat oven (**10.22**) operates by circulating air at a steady temperature of 190°C. An internal fan circulates the air over a heating element, through the instrument load, and back to the heater. At this temperature most *metal* instruments are not damaged.[20]

Studies have shown that it is possible to sterilise unwrapped instruments in 6 minutes, and wrapped instruments in 12 minutes.[21]

The load size of this steriliser is comparatively small.

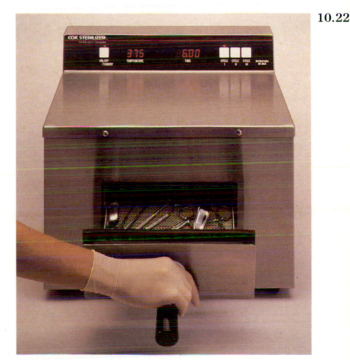

10.22

10.22   The Cox rapid heat transfer steriliser. (Courtesy Cox Sterile Products Ltd.)

Hot bead/salt sterilisers

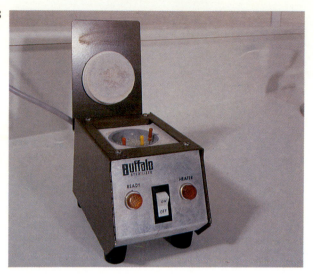

10.23

10.23 The glass bead steriliser.

Glass bead/salt sterilisers (**10.23**) are useful for sterilising small instruments such as endodontic files and rotary instruments. The steriliser is essentially a metal cup (crucible) in which the medium is maintained at 218–246°C. It is useful for sterilising endodontic files *during* endodontic treatment of multirooted teeth, to prevent transfer of infection between canals.

A minimum of 15 seconds immersion is recommended for effective sterilisation,[22] but the manufacturer's instructions should be followed, and instruments to be sterilised should be *thoroughly* clean.

Hot salt sterilisers are preferable to glass bead sterilisers for endodontic therapy. Residual salt or glass beads on the surface of the sterile endodontic instruments can cause blockage of the root canals. If salt granules are the cause of the blockage, they can be dissolved with irrigation.[23,24]

A suitable thermometer should be routinely used to ensure that the temperature reaches 218°C, as the temperature of the medium at the centre of the steriliser may be lower than that at the sides of the container.

Chemical 'sterilisation'

See Chapter 8.

Monitoring sterilisation

Recent studies[25] have described a 51% sterilisation failure rate in dental sterilisers. Other studies also indicate a high sterilisation failure rate when dental sterilisers were tested.[26,27]

It is evident that an alarming number of dental office sterilisers are not effective in killing all the spores present in biological indicators.

Variables, such as loading and wrapping of instruments, maintenance, cleaning, operating temperature, and exposure time, all affect the efficiency of the steriliser.

Heat sterilisation is the only decontamination process that can be easily and reliably checked to see that it works. There are two types of test:

Tests using chemical indicators

Test strips or tubes are available for autoclaves, chemiclaves, and dry-heat ovens; these should be used as recommended by the manufacturer. Chemical indicators show that sterilising conditions have been reached *not* that sterilisation has occurred. However, they are *very* useful for early detection of problems.

Several types of colour-change strips or tapes indicate temperature change only, that is, they *only* show that the load has been in a heat steriliser.

Superior colour-change indicators are available which are sensitive to both temperature and time. TST strips available in the UK and USA (**10.24**) monitor temperature and time during an autoclave cycle. Chemical indicators are placed in an open tray to monitor each processing cycle, and in *every* pack, pouch, or lidded tray.

Check that the indicator used is suitable for the steriliser. If the correct colour change does not occur, test using a microbiological indicator.

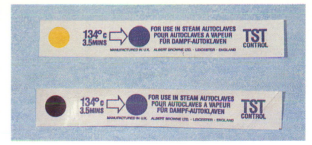

10.24   TST strip before and after processing.

Biological monitors

The routine *weekly* use of biological indicators (spore tests) to verify the adequacy of sterilisation cycles is recommended by the American Dental Association (ADA) and the Centers for Disease Control (CDC). Biological indicators (**10.25, 10.26**) verify the actual killing of bacterial spores used in the indicators, and therefore monitor actual sterilisation.

Procedure

Check with the manufacturer of the steriliser, to obtain the correct spore test. *Bacillus stearothermophilus* is used for chemical vapour and steam sterilisers, and *B. subtilis* is used for dry-heat spore testing. Put the correct type of test spores inside a pack, or near the centre of a typical load.

Mail the exposed test spores to an appropriate sterilisation monitoring service. A list of products and services is available from the Council on Dental Therapeutics. In all monitoring, a biological indicator which has not been exposed to the sterilisation process should be cultured to provide a control. Some strips and vials are available which may be cultured in the dental office. It has been demonstrated that both *B. subtilis* and *B. stearothermophilus* show a 90% reduction in growth during incubation, when stored at room temperature for 48 hours after sub-lethal exposure to a sterilisation agent.[28] This reduction could possibly take place in the mail during transit of the monitor, giving a false negative, result. To reduce these false negatives, incubation must begin shortly after sterilisation. Intra-office biological monitoring is highly recommended.

A positive culture result indicates that not all the spores were killed and the items processed in that load may not be sterile.

Positive results may be caused when:

- Packs are improperly prepared.
- The steriliser is improperly loaded.
- The steriliser does not work properly.
- The process time is too short.

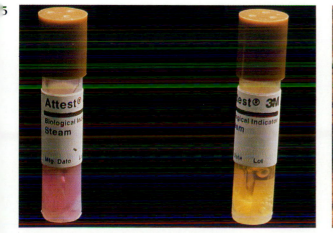

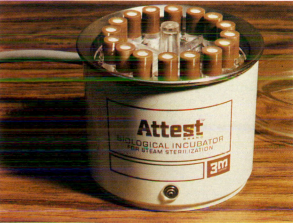

10.25   Negative (left) and positive (right) results with a biological indicator. (Courtesy 3M Health Care Ltd.)

10.26   A water-bath incubator, which can be used in a dental office. (Courtesy 3M Health Care Ltd.)

If a result is positive, repeat the spore test. Examine the procedures used, to check that:

- The steriliser is properly loaded and *not* overfilled.
- The packs are not too large.
- The manufacturer's instructions are followed.

If the result is positive a second time, do not use the steriliser until it has been inspected and repaired, or until the *exact* reason for the positive tests has been found. Reprocess any stored items which were sterilised after the last negative spore test.

The dental team should have *written* instructions for all decontamination procedures. Periodically, compare the technique used with the written instructions.

A record of weekly spore test results should be kept. A log of sterilisation tests (**10.27**) is used.

Chemical and biological monitors should be stored in a cool, dry place, and should not be used after the recommended expiry date.

Products

The following monitors were recommended by the CRA in 1986.[29]

Chemical vapour steriliser: Attest flash monitor. *Note:* A later CRA report[30] issued a warning that this monitor *should not* be used with the Harvey chemiclave, however these monitors have now been modified.

Autoclaves: Attest monitor.

Dry-heat sterilisers: Spordi monitor.

Log of microbiological monitor tests

Date of test
Steriliser model
Results
Action taken/comments

10.27   Log of spore test results: items to be included.

Special Considerations in Sterilisation and Disinfection

Most critical and semi-critical instruments can be sterilised by heat, but certain vital instruments which require heat sterilisation are damaged after repeated sterilisation cycles.

Dental handpieces

Contamination

During use, dental handpieces become contaminated with blood and saliva.[31,32] A handpiece may become contaminated in two ways:

Direct contact with blood, saliva, and other debris
During use, the external surfaces of the handpiece become contaminated. Blood and other tissue fluids may also enter the cartridge chamber around the bur mounting, causing internal contamination.

Water retraction
Water-retraction valves within dental units aspirate infective material back into the handpiece and water line (**10.28**). Water retraction is eliminated by fitting check valves to reduce the risk of transfer of infective material (**10.29**).

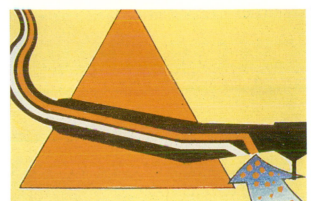

10.28 Water aspiration into a handpiece. (Courtesy Castellini Ltd.)

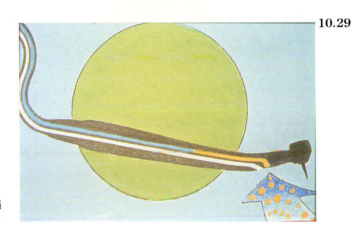

10.29

10.29 Minimising water retraction. (Courtesy Castellini Ltd.)

Current guidelines

UK

British Dental Association (BDA) and DOH guidelines state that handpieces should be sterilised in an autoclave between patients.

USA

The current CDC guideline recommends routine sterilisation of handpieces between patients, but recognises that not all handpieces can be sterilised. If a handpiece cannot be sterilised, it should be flushed, cleaned, and then disinfected using a chemical disinfectant that is registered with the EPA as a hospital disinfectant and is mycobacterial at use-dilution.

Many older or inferior types of current handpieces cannot be sterilised by heat without damage, such as degradation of fibre-optic bundles. This results in decreased light output, noise increase, early failure of bearing cages and bearings, and a need for increased air pressure.[33] Such damage usually occurs 3–9 months after routine sterilisation. Other experimental sterilisation techniques for the treatment of handpieces are being tested, e.g. a plasma steriliser that will sterilise a handpiece in 3–5 minutes without the use of heat.

Sterilisation of handpieces

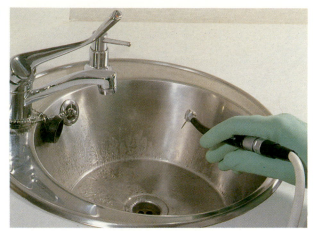

10.30

10.30   Run the handpiece over a sink.

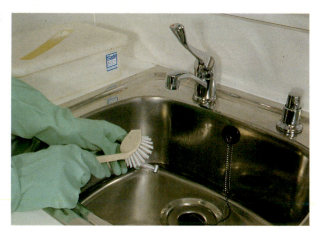

10.31

10.31   Scrub the handpiece thoroughly.

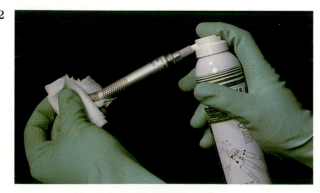

10.32

10.32   Lubricate the handpiece.

10.33   Expel excess oil, by hanging the handpiece in a rack.

Choose a good-quality handpiece capable of being sterilised by an autoclave or a chemiclave. Obtain a *written* guarantee from the manufacturer or supplier that the handpiece may be sterilised without damage over a reasonable period of time. Follow the manufacturer's cleaning, lubrication, and sterilisation instructions *exactly*.

The following routine illustrates the basic stages of handpiece sterilisation, these stages may differ for different makes of handpiece.

- Run the handpiece over a sink for 20 seconds allowing water to flush through the handpiece thoroughly (**10.30**). Remove the bur.
- Scrub the handpiece thoroughly (**10.31**) with a detergent and water, to remove any debris. Rinse and dry the handpiece.
- Lubricate the handpiece with a good quality oil recommended by the handpiece manufacturer (**10.32**).
- Expel excess oil by running the handpiece for 20 seconds, after replacing the bur or hanging the handpiece in a handpiece rack (**10.33**).
- Remove the bur, if replaced. Clean the fibre-optic bundle ends with alcohol (**10.34**).
- Place the handpiece in a clearview sterilisation pouch, together with a chemical indicator strip (**10.35**).
- Sterilise in an autoclave or chemiclave, according to the manufacturer's instructions (**10.36**). Do not leave the handpiece in the steriliser after the sterilisation cycle is complete.
- Remove the handpiece from the bag, insert the bur, and use.

Note: Some makes of handpieces require relubrication *after* sterilisation, e.g. Midwest handpieces. Consult the handpiece manufacturer. If relubrication after sterilisation is necessary, a separate clean oil-spray container should be used, to prevent recontamination.

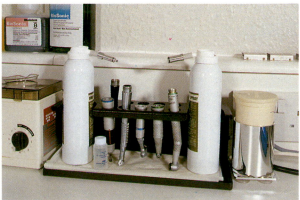

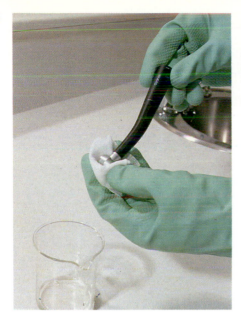

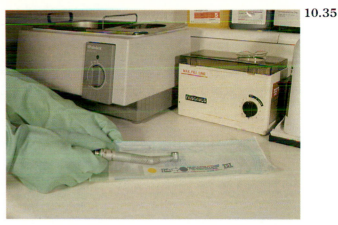

10.35 Place the handpiece in a clearview sterilisation pouch.

10.34 Clean the fibre-optic ends with alcohol.

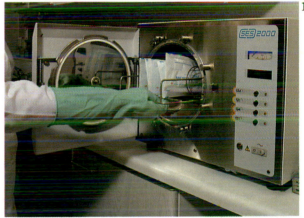

Precautions

Conventional dry heat cannot be used on any turbine handpiece currently sold.[33] Repeated lubrication followed by heat sterilisation can cause lubricant build-up, resulting in sluggish performance. Manufacturers should consider producing solvents which remove old lubricant prior to relubrication.[33] Use the lubricant recommended by the manufacturer.

10.36 Sterilise the handpiece.

Do not operate a handpiece without a bur. Do not sterilise a handpiece with the bur installed.

The CRA (November 1990) report tested the Kavoclave (Supraclave) (10.37) and recommended its use for the sterilisation of handpieces using low heat (121°C) and steam under pressure.

Modern turbine handpieces are being introduced which withstand repeated heat sterilisation. The new Kavo range of handpieces, for example, have solid fibre-optic rods instead of fibre-optic bundles and new heat-resistant cartridges. Another development is the introduction of ceramic bearings by the Den-Tal-E3 Star Company. Also, lubrication-free handpieces, such as the 430 SWL Lube-free handpiece, may be resistant to damage from repeated sterilisation cycles, and are being tested by the CRA in the USA.

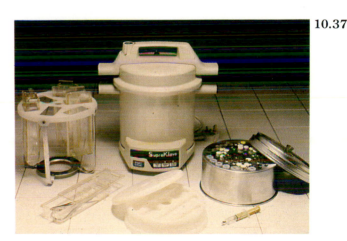

10.37 The Supraclave.

The number of handpieces required

Plan *one hour* to prepare, sterilise, and cool a handpiece.[33] Use the general formulae below, to determine the number of handpieces required per surgery.

One patient treated per hour—2 of each type of handpiece.

Two patients treated per hour—3 of each type of handpiece.

Handpiece disinfection

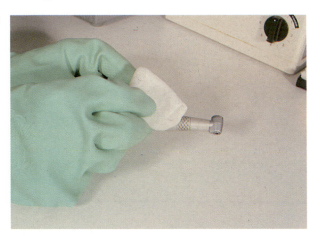

10.38 Wipe the handpiece with an EPA-registered disinfectant.

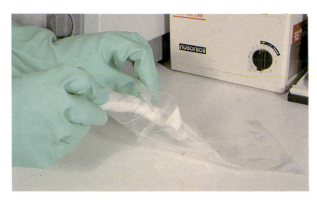

10.39 Wrap in saturated, absorbent material and cover with a plastic wrap.

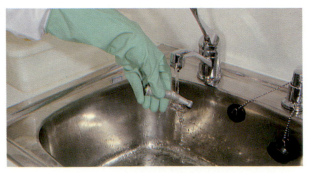

If a handpiece *cannot* be sterilised it should be disinfected between patients. This procedure is a compromise and is *not* high-level disinfection. At best, it is intermediate level. The inside of the handpiece which may be heavily contaminated is *not* disinfected.

Prolonged use of disinfectants will damage certain metal handpiece alloys and chucking mechanisms. Some manufacturers of handpieces do not recommend this method and this could make the product warranty void. Crevices and joints of the dental handpieces may preclude consistent surface disinfection, regardless of the anti-microbial activity of the disinfectant.[34]

Procedure

Important: *The procedure described is used on handpieces that cannot be sterilised. A dentist should purchase handpieces capable of being sterilised using an autoclave or a chemiclave as soon as possible.*

- Flush the handpiece thoroughly with water for 20 seconds.
- Scrub the handpiece with water to remove debris.
- *Wipe* the handpiece with a clean, absorbent material saturated with an EPA-registered tuberculocidal disinfectant. Wet the surfaces thoroughly with the disinfectant (**10.38**).
- Keep the handpiece wet for the time stated on the disinfectant label (usually 10 minutes) by wrapping it in saturated, absorbent material and covering with a plastic wrap (**10.39**).
- Rinse the handpiece thoroughly with water, to remove chemical residues which may irritate hands or harm patients (**10.40**).

10.40 Rinse the handpiece thoroughly.

The turbonet system

The turbonet system is a device which disinfects and thoroughly cleans handpieces (**10.41**).[35]

It has been found that if glutaraldehyde phenate (sporicidin) is used in this device, it will corrode turbine component parts made from aluminium.[36] Practitioners should consult the handpiece manufacturer before using the turbonet system. This system does not sterilise handpieces.

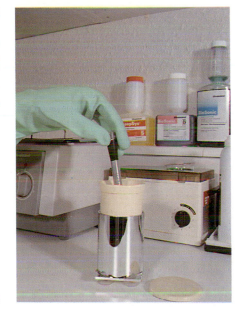

10.41 The turbonet system.

Decident disposable disinfectant sleeve

The decident sleeve is a laminated metallised pouch (**10.42**). It contains a foam liner soaked with disinfectant (67% w/w ethyl alcohol, 0.5% *p*-tert amylphenol, 0.2% *o*-phenylphenol, and corrosion inhibitors).

It is used to provide *maximum* contact of the disinfectant with a handpiece (**10.42**) for the recommended time (10 minutes) (**10.43**).

The disinfectant has excellent antimicrobial activity.[37] Careful attention must be given to each step of the instructions.

The disinfectant has been found to damage the chuck in auto-chuck, push-button, and latch handpieces, rendering them incapable of retaining burs. Low-speed and high-speed handpieces, using bur changers, are not adversely affected.[37] This system does *not* sterilise handpieces.

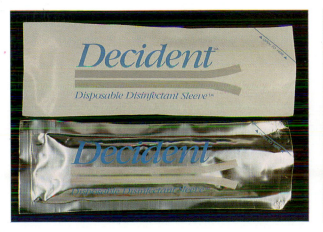

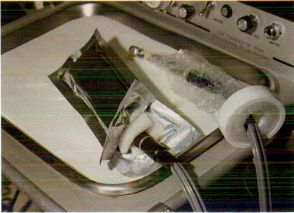

10.42 The decident sleeve. (Courtesy Dr J. Young, University of Texas.)

10.43 The decident sleeve in use. (Courtesy Dr J. Young, University of Texas.)

Rotary instruments

Burs become very contaminated and are classed as critical items; they must be sterilised after use.

Diamond and carbide burs may be safely autoclaved with minimal damage[38] but carbon-steel burs are damaged by autoclaving.

Carbon-steel burs may be sterilised by using a chemical vapour steriliser. A glass bead steriliser at 218°C for 10 seconds may be used to sterilise grossly contaminated carbon-steel burs during the same dental procedure.[38]

Some polishing stones and composite finishing stones are damaged by heat sterilisation. Before considering sterilisation of stones and other rotary polishing instruments, consult the manufacturer's instructions.

Retentive pin-twist drills may be sterilised by the steam autoclave or the chemical vapour steriliser with minimal effect on the mean fracture strength,[39] but it has been found that sterilisation using a steam autoclave reduces the cutting efficiency of retentive pin-twist drills.

The amalgam carrier

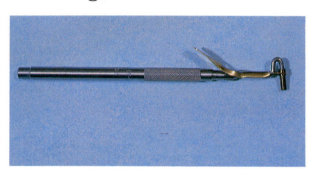

10.44 External-spring mechanism amalgam carrier. (Courtesy Hu Friedy, USA.)

The dental amalgam carrier becomes very contaminated, especially around the external and internal surface of the tip.[40]

Many amalgam carriers cannot be autoclaved without damage, and studies have shown that immersion in a 1% glutaraldehyde disinfectant for 10 minutes was only 75% effective against common oral bacteria.[40]

It is recommended that amalgam carriers should be sterilised using heat sterilisation. Practitioners should consider purchasing amalgam carriers capable of withstanding heat sterilisation without damage. It has been found that external-spring mechanism amalgam carriers (**10.44**) can be effectively sterilised by autoclaving.[40]

Visible-light curing units

It has been shown that light curing devices are a potential source of transmission of infectious diseases, due to contamination of the light curing tip, which directly contacts oral structures, and the handle, which becomes contaminated with blood and saliva from the operator's or assistant's gloved hands.[41]

Some new designs of unit feature removable, autoclavable light curing tips. However, the handles still present a problem, since they cannot be sterilised.

Units should be cleaned and disinfected with a phenolic disinfectant after use.[42] Plastic units should be disinfected using an iodophor. Glutaraldehyde disinfectants have been found to damage the glass rods in a fibre-optic light tip, with a subsequent reduction in light output; the use of this disinfectant should be avoided.[43]

Procedure

Thoroughly wipe and clean the whole unit. If the fibre-optic light tip can be sterilised, detach it and sterilise as recommended by the manufacturer. Wrap the handle and light curing tip (if not autoclavable) in a wrap, soaked with an iodophore disinfectant (**10.45**). The wrap should remain in place for at least 10 minutes or until the unit is next used. Remove the wrap and wipe the unit with distilled water to remove residual disinfectant.

Some practitioners cover the top light curing tip with clingfilm (**10.46**), which is removed after use. This appears to have minimal effect on the curing effectiveness of the unit, and protects the curing tip from blood, saliva, and other debris.

Disposable protective coverings could be used on the handles, providing they do not interfere with the unit's cooling mechanism.

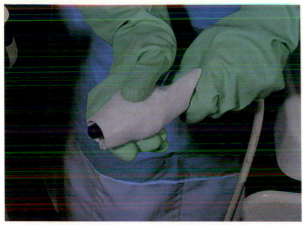

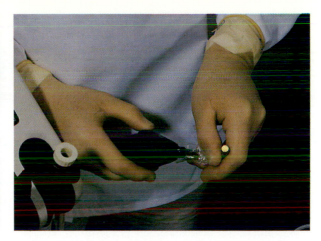

10.45 Wrap the handle and light curing tip in a wrap soaked with disinfectant.

10.46 Covering the top light curing tip with clingfilm.

Anaesthetic equipment

Several studies[44,45] describe extensive contamination of anaesthetic masks after use. However, there is limited evidence of cross contamination from anaesthetic equipment.[45]

Dentists should be familiar with recommendations from the Royal College of Anaesthetists (UK) and from the American College of Anaesthesiology (USA).

Disinfection procedure

- Scrub masks and hoses with detergent and water.
- Disinfect masks and hoses by immersion in 1:213 iodophor for 10 minutes.
- Thoroughly rinse under tap water to remove all residual disinfectant.

Nitrous-oxide masks and anaesthetic hoses which can be heat-sterilised are available.

References

[1] Simpson, J. P. and Whitaker, D. K. Serum contamination of instruments in dental practice. *Br. Dent. J.*, 1979; **146**:76–8.

[2] Eames, W. B., Bryington, S. Q., Sunway, N. B. A comparison of eight ultrasonic cleaners. *Gen. Dent.*, 1982; **30**:242–5.

[3] Palenik, F. J. and Miller, C. H. In vitro testing of three dental cleaning systems. *J. Prosth. Dent.*, 1984; **51**:751–4.

[4] Matis, B. A. et al. Aeromedical Review. *Ultrasonic cleaners*. USAF School of Aerospace – Medical Books Air Force Base 1982. Review 1–82.

[5] Sandford, J. E. Cleaning with ultrasonics. *Amer. Machinist.*, 1966; **110**:87–98.

[6] Miller, C. H. and Hardwick, L. M. Ultrasonic cleaning of dental instruments in cassettes. *Gen. Dent.*, 1988; **36**:31–6.

[7] Napier, B. W. D. and Senotore, R. U. They do clean burs don't they? *J. Dent. Assoc.*, 1988; **43**:585.

[8] Patterson, C. J. W., McLundie, A. C., McKay, A. M. The effect of ultrasonic cleaning and autoclaving on tungsten carbide burs. *Br. Dent. J.*, 1988; **164**:113–15.

[9] Clinical Research Associates. Report, August 1989; **13**(8).

[10] Department of Health. HE1 200, HMSO, October 1990.

[11] Department of Health. HE1 185, HMSO, July 1988.

[12] Department of Health. HE1 196, HMSO, March 1990.

[13] Health & Safety Executive. *Safety of Autoclaves,* Guidance note PM73, HMSO, 1990.

[14] Wood, P. R. and Martin, M. V. A study of autoclave bags in non-vacuum autoclaves. *J. Dent.*, 1987; **17**:148–9.

[15] Bertolotti, R. L. and Hurst, V. Inhibition of corrosion during autoclave sterilization of carbon steel dental instruments. *J. Am. Dent. Assoc.*, 1978; **97**:628–32.

[16] Johnson, G. K., Perry, F. V., Pelleu, G. B. Effect of four anticorrosive dips on the cutting efficiency of dental carbide burs. *J. Am. Dent. Assoc.*, 1987; **114**:648–50.

[17] US Dept. of Labor. Occupational Safety and Health Administration. *Occupational exposure to formaldehyde; Final Rule.* Fed. Reg. 1987; **52**:168–312.

[18] Ko, S. S., Quale, A. A., Rothwell, P. S. Basic performance and production load testing of hot air sterilizers for use in dental surgeries. *J. Dent.*, 1987; **15**:178–80.

[19]American Dental Association. Monograph series on Dental materials and Therapeutics: *Safety and Infection Control in the Dental Office;* First edition, 1990; 47–9.

[20]Kolstad, R. A. Rapid dry heat sterilization. *J. Clin. Orth.,* 1988;**22(12)**:768–9.

[21]Clinical Research Associates Newsletter. *Sterilizer, Dry heat (circulated air).* 1989;**13(9)**:2–3.

[22]Dayoub, M. B. and Devine, M. J. Endodontic dry heat sterilizers. *J. Endod.,* 1976;**2**:343–4.

[23]Grossman, L. I. *Endodontic practice,* 9th edn., Philadelphia: Lea and Febiger, 1978: 165.

[24]Weine, F. S. *Endodontic therapy,* 2nd edn., St. Louis., C. V. Mosby Co., 1976:416.

[25]Nickerson, A., Bhuta, P., Orton, G., Alvin, B. Monitoring dental sterilizers. Effectiveness using biological indicators. *J. Dent. Hyg.,* 1990;**64**:69–73.

[26]Simonsen, R. J., Schachtele, C. F., Joos, R. W. An evaluation of sterilization by autoclave in dental offices. *J. Dent. Res.,* 1979;**58** (Special issue A): 1–6.

[27]Christensen, R. P. and Christen, J. H. Evaluation of an autoclave monitoring system. *J. Dent. Res.,* 1980;**59** (Special issue A) Abstract: 391.

[28]Caputo, R. A., Rohn, K. J., Mascoli, C. C. Recovery of biological organisms after sterilization treatment. *J. Parenter. Drug Assoc.,* 1980;**34**:394–7.

[29]Clinical Research Associates, Newsletter. Sept. 1986; **10(9)**.

[30]Clinical Research Associates, Newsletter. Feb. 1988; **12(2)**.

[31]Kellet, M., Holbrook, W. P. Bacterial contamination of dental handpieces. *J. Dent.,* 1980;**8**:249–53.

[32]Bond, M. S. Viral hepatitis safety in the immuno chemistry laboratory. *Liq. and Qlty.,* 1982;**5**:1, 34–9.

[33]Clinical Research Associates, Newsletter. Handpieces, sterilization disinfection. *Oral Health,* 1988;**78(8)**:29–32.

[34]Robinson, D., Robinson, R., Christensen, R. Disinfection of dental handpieces. *J. Dent. Res.,* 1990;**69**:348–9.

[35]Oluwole, A., Stupart, B., Boyd, J., Siguenza, R., Sinkford, J. Efficacy of glutaraldehyde-phenate as a disinfecting agent for high speed handpieces. *Quint. Int.,* 1989;**20**:637–40.

[36]Oluwole, A. Boyd, J., Siguenza, A., Sinkford, J. Scannery electron microscopic evaluation of the micro-corrosive effect of alkaline glutaraldehyde-phenate on a high speed turbine. *Quint. Int.,* 1989;**20**:265–9.

[37]Clinical Research Associates, Newsletter. Subject: *Disinfection of handpieces,* 1990;**14(4)**:1–2.

[38]McDonnell, C. J., Baumgarter, J. C., Vermilyea, S. G. Durability of dental burs following multiple sterilization cycles. *Gen. Dent.,* 1989;**37(6)**:485–9.

[39]Cooley, R., Marshall, T., Young, J., Huddleston, A. Effect of sterilization on the strength and cutting efficiency of twist drills. *Quint. Int.,* 1990;**21**:919–23.

[40]Schwass, D. R., Stokes, A. N., Sutherland, A. P., Hood, J. A. Effectiveness of sterilization and disinfection procedures for dental amalgam carriers. *N. Z. Dent. J.,* 1990;**86**:62–4.

[41]Caughman, W., O'Connor, R. P., Volkmann, K. R., Schuster, G. S., Caughman, G. B. Visible light curing devices a potential source of disease transmission. *Operative Dentistry,* 1987;**12**:10–14.

[42]Caughman, G. B., Caughman, W. F., Napier, N., Schuster, G. S. Disinfection of visible-light curing devices. *Operative Dentistry,* 1989;**14**:2–7.

[43]Dugan, W. T. and Hartleb, J. H. Influence of a glutaraldehyde disinfecting solution on curing light effectiveness. *Gen. Dent.,* 1989;**40(3)**:40–43.

[44]Yagiela, Y. A., Hunt, L. M., Hunt, D. Disinfection of nitrous oxide inhalation equipment. *J. Am. Dent. Assoc.,* 1979;**98**:191–5.

[45]Hunt, L. M. and Yagiela, J. A. Bacterial contamination and transmission by nitrous oxide sedation apparatus. *Oral Surg.,* 1977;**44**:367–73.

11. Dental Equipment

The Dental Unit, Chair, and Cabinetry Design

It is difficult to clean and disinfect the surfaces of older dental equipment (**11.1, 11.2**). External surfaces of suction tubing and water/air outlet tubing are corrugated, and in some cases covered in fabric. Switches on older dental units are not easy to disinfect and the constant application of disinfectant solutions may cause damage. Dental chairs may be covered in fabric, or the covering material and stitching have become damaged by long-term application of disinfectant solutions.

Because of the damage caused to the surfaces and controls of older dental equipment, the practitioner may prefer to cover certain surfaces rather than apply disinfectant solutions.

Manufacturers are now producing dental equipment of the highest standard which can be cleaned and disinfected easily with minimal damage.

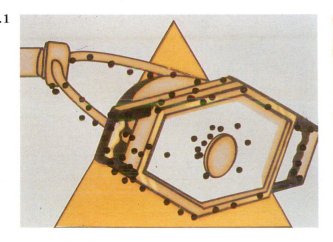

11.1 Contamination of the surface of a lamp. (Courtesy Castellini.)

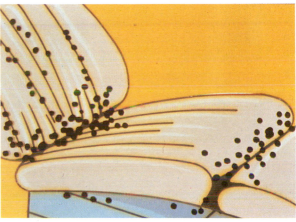

11.2 Contamination of the dental chair. (Courtesy Castellini.)

Points to consider when purchasing a unit

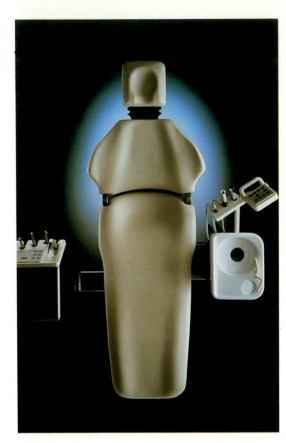

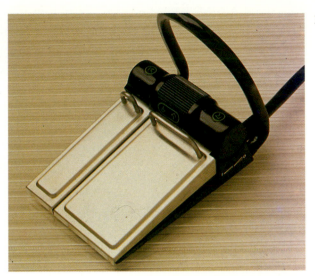

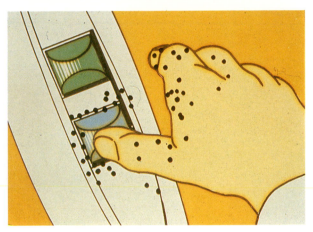

11.3 Chairs are available with seamless surfaces that are easy to disinfect. Chair arms become very contaminated and are difficult to clean and disinfect (especially the arm near the spittoon). Many new models do not have arms. (Courtesy Siemens.)

11.4, 11.5 Certain models of chair have foot controls, eliminating the need to disinfect hand-operated chair control switches. (Courtesy Castellini.)

11.6

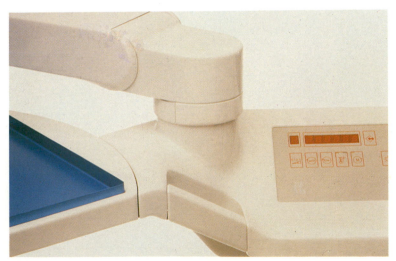

11.6 Handles, e.g. bracket table handles, are smooth and easily cleaned. Some can be detached and are autoclavable. (Courtesy Kavo.)

11.7

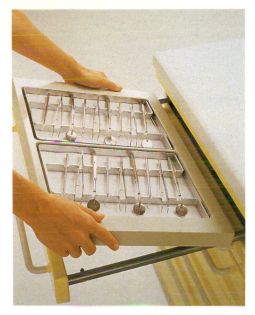

11.8

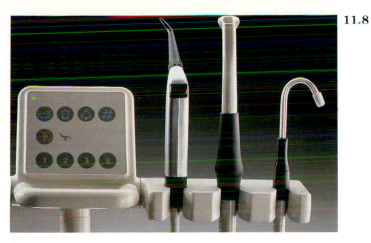

11.8 Controls are covered with membranes and are easy to clean. (Courtesy Siemens.)

11.7 Cabinets should have smooth surfaces with rounded corners. In some cases, drawer and shelf interiors can be removed and cleaned. (Courtesy Siemens.)

9

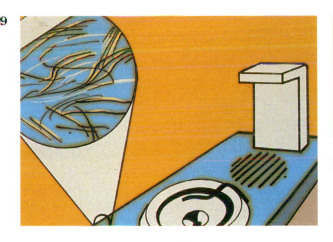

11.10

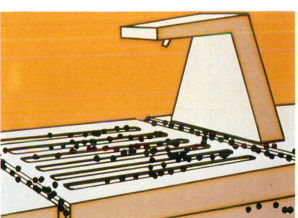

11.9–11.11 If the outer surface and surrounding area of the spittoon are easily scratched, they become difficult to clean and disinfect (**11.9**). Sharp angles and corners should be avoided in these areas (**11.10**). Modern units use a *single* piece of vitreous china, which is resistant to abrasion (**11.11**). (Courtesy Castellini.)

11.11

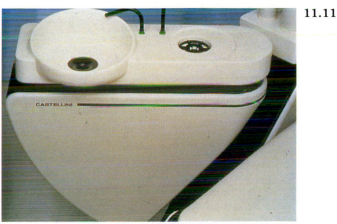

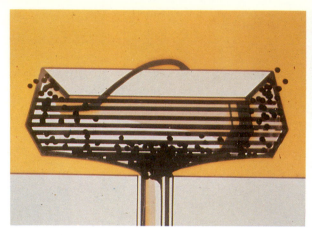
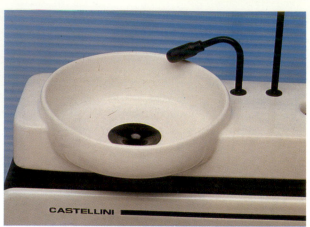

11.12, 11.13 When the tube that supplies water to the spittoon is below the rim, there is a risk of contact between the contaminated water in the spittoon and the water in the unit supply if the drain becomes blocked (**11.12**). Modern units position the tube that supplies water to the spittoon at a level above the rim (**11.13**). Some units provide a constant supply of disinfectant to the spittoon. (Courtesy Castellini.)

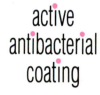
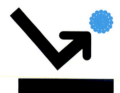
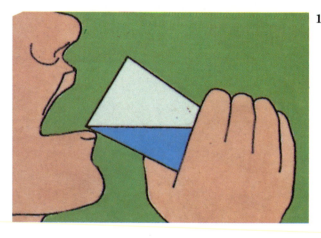

11.14 Some dental units have surfaces which they claim do not provide an environment favourable to the proliferation of bacteria. Such surface coatings are said to contain anti-microbial agents. (Courtesy Castellini.)

11.15 Automatic disinfectant dispensers add chlorhexidine to the water supplied to the mouthwash cup (Courtesy Castellini.)

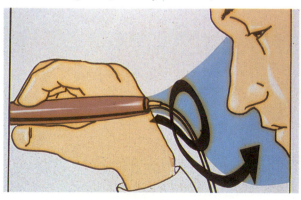
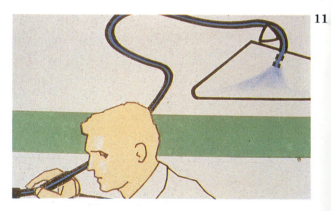

11.16 Contaminated escaping air is discharged near the face of the operator, when the turbine is used with two- or three-way connections. (Courtesy Castellini.)

11.17 Four-way couplings fitted to air-operated instruments allow air to escape from the turbine, away from the operator. (Courtesy Castellini.)

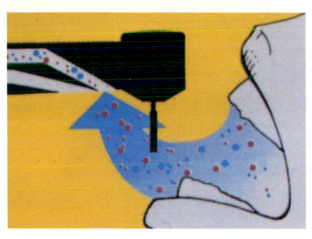

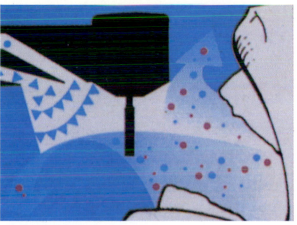

11.18, 11.19   Water retraction is prevented mainly by fitting anti-retraction valves. One manufacturer prevents the re-aspiration of the spray (**11.18**) by minimising re-aspiration at the turbine head (**11.19**). This should be used in conjunction with anti-retraction valves. (Courtesy Castellini.)

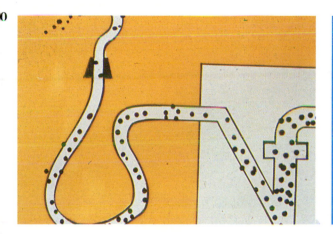

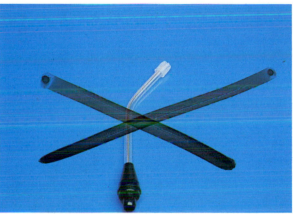

11.20, 11.21   'Venturi effect' saliva ejectors, create a confluence of the contaminated line with the drinking water line (**11.20**). Some units have a system of water-flow inversion to clean the filter. Such a system can cause contamination of the dental unit water supply. Newer dental units do not use this system (**11.21**). (Courtesy Castellini.)

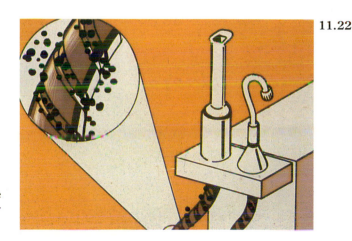

11.22   The aspirator-tip holder, the filter box, and the aspiration tubes with corrugations, all become very contaminated. (Courtesy Castellini.)

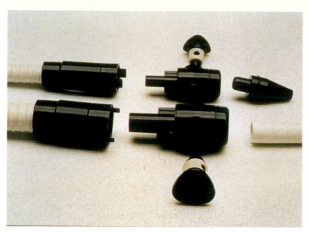

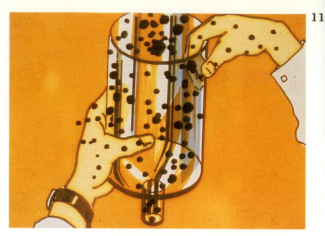

11.23   Manufacturers have made the aspirator-tip holder and filter box easily detachable and autoclavable. Aspirator tubes should have both external and internal surfaces as smooth as possible without any fluting. Some tubes are detachable, allowing periodic higher-level disinfection. (Courtesy Castellini.)

11.24   The separation bowl (linked to the spittoon and suction) becomes very contaminated and requires frequent cleaning. This procedure places the dental assistant in direct contact with high-risk infection zones. (Courtesy Castellini.)

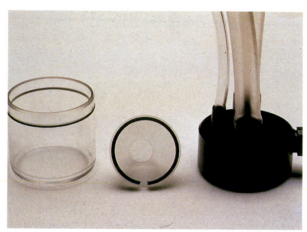

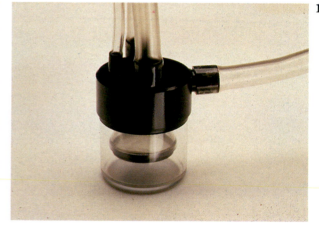

11.25, 11.26   The solid waste separating bowl causes the sedimentation of solids (especially amalgam), thus separating them from the water outlet flow. This system should very efficiently reduce pollution and is easy to clean. (Courtesy Castellini.)

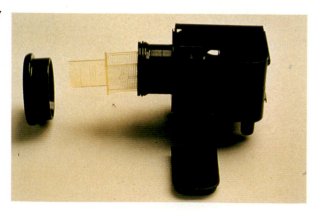

11.27   Certain units supply a constant emission of non-foaming disinfectant detergent from a unit that is linked to the aspiration system. (Courtesy Castellini.)

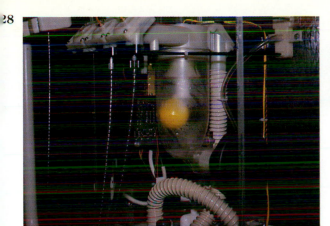

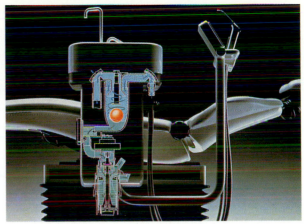

11.28, 11.29 Advanced solid waste separating systems are available on some units. These are not only very efficient, but require minimal cleaning and maintenance. (Courtesy Siemens.)

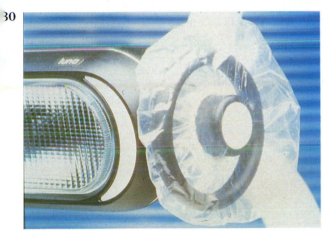

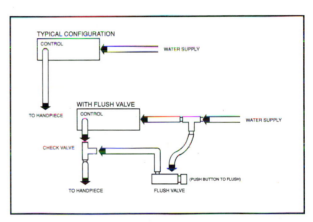

11.30 A variety of covers which are tailor-made for chair head rests, handles, bracket tables water line tubing, etc. are available from dental distributors. (Courtesy Castellini.)

11.31 Before reuse, handpieces and water line tubing must be effectively flushed to remove contaminated water. A kit is available which can be added to any make of dental unit. This flushes an increased volume of water through water lines and reduces flush time to 5 seconds. This is accomplished without running the handpiece and causing more aerosol spray. (Courtesy Adec.)

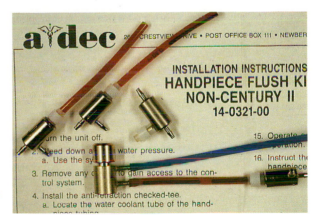

11.32 The kit that is available from Adec, also contains anti-retraction valves. (Courtesy Adec and Dr J.M. Young.)

The Dental Unit Water Supply

There is ample evidence that the dental unit water supply is contaminated with micro-organisms,[1-8] such as, pseudomonas, haemolytic streptococci, non-haemolytic streptococci, and enterococci.[1]

Until fairly recently, the transmission of infection from the dental unit water supply was considered only theoretical. However, one report[9] describes infection of medically compromised patients by *Pseudomonas aeruginosa*, which originated from the dental unit water supply. The same study found that infections were not established in non-medically compromised patients.

Contamination of the dental unit water supply originates from three sources:

- Many older units are fitted with retraction valves. These aspirate water that has been contaminated with oral micro-organisms into the dental unit water lines.[1,2,5]
- Air/water syringes, turbines, and ultrasonic scalers become internally contaminated by oral micro-organisms during use. Passive retraction from these instruments, causing contamination of dental unit water lines, is possible.[2,4,5,10]
- Bacteria already present in tap water may contaminate the dental unit water supply.[1,6,7,11]

Once micro-organisms have gained access to the unit water supply, they are capable of colonising, multiplying, and contaminating water in the dental unit. They may be a constant source of contaminated discharge from the turbine, air/water syringe, and ultrasonic scaler.[1,2,4,5,10]

Precautions to minimise contamination

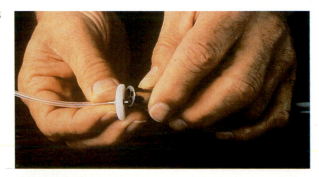

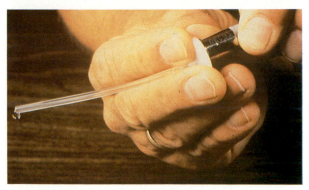

11.33, 11.34 Water retraction test kit from Adec. (Courtesy Dr J.J. Crawford.)

1. A dental unit may be tested to determine the degree of water retraction by using a simple water retraction test kit available from Adec[5] (**11.33, 11.34**).

   Retraction of oral micro-organisms into turbine hoses occurs in *uncorrected* units fitted with a retraction valve.[5] This has been demonstrated by using red dye (**11.35**)[5] It is possible to aspirate 1 ml of contaminated water into the dental unit water line.[2] Fitting a non-retraction valve will partially prevent contamination of the dental unit water supply.[2,5]

   A check or non-retraction valve reduces contamination of dental unit water lines but does not eliminate colonisation of the dental unit water supply by aquatic bacteria already present in tap water or prevent passive spread of micro-organisms from the turbine, air/water syringe, or ultrasonic scaler.[2,4,5,10]

   A kit is available from Adec which includes check valves capable of being fitted to most makes of dental units.[5] Information supplied by manufacturers on current makes of dental units and their retraction status has been published by the American Dental Association (ADA).[12]

   Aspirated oral bacteria may be expelled into the mouth of the next patient and may also colonise water lines in the dental unit.[2]

2. Fitting a sterile turbine handpiece, a sterile air/water syringe, or a sterile ultrasonic scaler after each treatment, reduces but does not totally eliminate the discharge of contaminated water.[1–4,7]

3. Flushing the air/water lines between patients for 20 seconds, then fitting a sterile turbine, sterile ultrasonic scaler tip, or sterile air water syringe tip *reduces* but does not completely eliminate the discharge of contaminated water from air lines.[4,5]

It has been recommended that air/water lines, which have stood unused overnight, should be flushed for 2 minutes before use.[4]

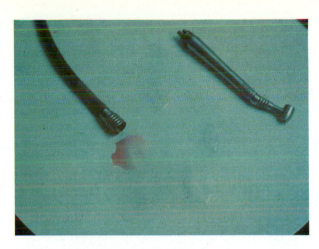

11.35

11.35 Retraction into turbine hoses, demonstrated by use of a red dye. (Courtesy Dr J.J. Crawford.)

Summary

A substantial, but not total, reduction in the level of contamination of the dental unit water supply and of the water discharged from the turbine handpiece, the air/water syringe, and the ultrasonic scaler can be achieved by:

- Fitting check or non-retraction valves to the dental unit.
- Fitting a sterile handpiece, a sterile air/water syringe (or tips), and a sterile ultrasonic scaler before treatment of the next patient.
- Flushing the air/water lines connected to the turbine handpiece, ultrasonic scaler, or air/water syringe between patients.

Disinfection of the Dental Unit Water Supply

Further reduction of contamination of the dental unit water supply can be achieved by disinfecting the water supply to or within the dental unit.

One study has underlined the difficulties faced when attempting disinfection of the dental unit water supply.[13] Micro-organisms are embedded in a biofilm attached to the internal surface of dental unit water lines. Disinfectants must remove the biofilm to achieve long-lasting disinfection. It was found that glutaraldehyde and free chlorine did not remove or destroy micro-organisms within the biofilm, however a solution of hydrogen peroxide was effective.

Despite this, hypochlorite and glutaraldehyde have been successfully used to disinfect the dental unit water supply,[3,6,8] but their residual action is of limited duration.

Several methods are available to maintain a fresh supply of clean, disinfected water from the dental unit:

- Povidone iodine 10% used for 24 hours to disinfect the unit water line, followed by the constant use of sterile water, prevented contamination of the dental unit water supply for 3–14 days.[3] Sterile water *alone* did not reduce the level of micro-organisms; preliminary disinfection is essential.

- Disinfection of the mains water which supplied the dental units was successfully achieved, by adding 15% sodium hypochlorite close to the main water intake for 10 minutes each day.[6]
- The Adec clean water reservoir may be fitted to any make of equipment (**11.36, 11.37**). Clinical research has shown that a weekly flush of 1% sodium hypochlorite will disinfect the dental unit water supply. Use of sterile water following the flush will provide a bacteria-free water system for a week.[8]
- Modern dental units are now available which have the facility to provide disinfected or sterile water to the air/water outlet tubes and to the water supplying the tumbler filler (**11.38–11.41**).
- A kit is available which determines the level of contamination of the dental unit water supply (**11.42–11.45**).

11.36

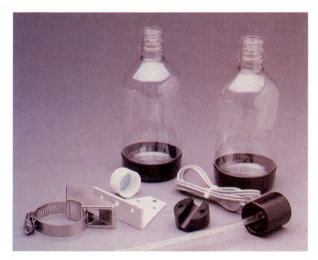

11.37

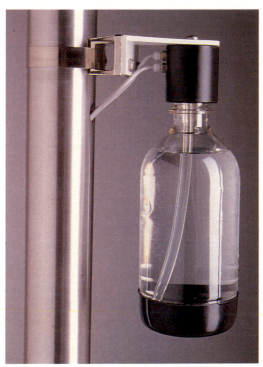

11.36, 11.37 The Adec clean water reservoir. (Courtesy Adec.)

11.38

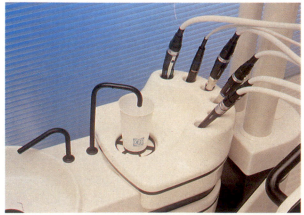

11

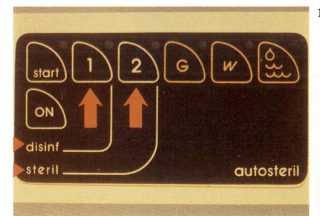

11.38, 11.39 The Castellini autosteril system. (Courtesy Castellini.)

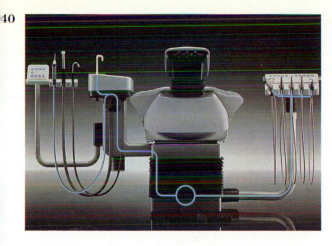

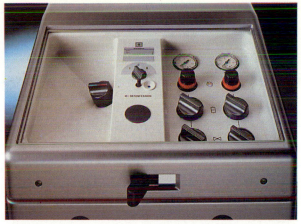

11.40 The Siemens disinfecting system. (Courtesy Siemens.)

11.41 Control box for the Siemens system in **11.40**, located in the chair base. (Courtesy Siemens.)

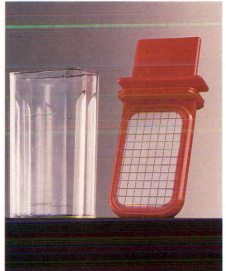

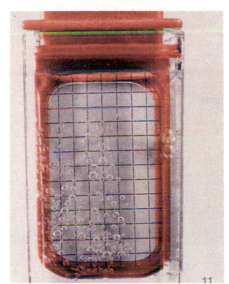

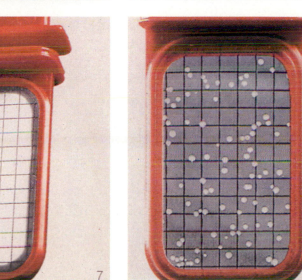

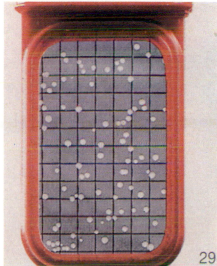

11.42–11.45 Kit to determine the level of contamination of the dental unit water supply. (Courtesy Siemens.)

Triple Syringe—Air/Water Syringe

11.46

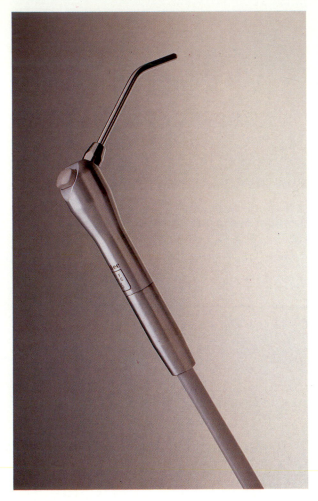

Air/water syringes have been found to be contaminated after use. The highest level of contamination is found within the lumen of the syringe tips, but the outside of the barrels may also be contaminated.[14] Reusing a contaminated air/water syringe may cause cross contamination. Syringes are available with easily detachable and autoclavable tips; or better still, fully autoclavable air/water syringes are available (**11.46**).

Many air/water syringes retract contaminated oral fluids into the syringe tip when the water valve is released.[14] The new Adec air/water syringe is *non-water retracting*.

Contamination of the dental unit water supply can occur from a contaminated air/water syringe.[4]

11.46 Adec autoclavable air/water syringe. (Courtesy Adec.)

Recommendations

11.47

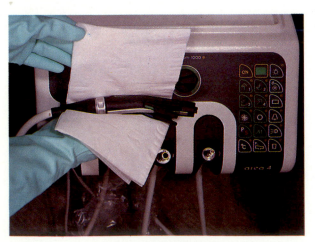

- Use an autoclavable non-water retracting air/water syringe.
- If this is not possible, use a sterile air/water syringe tip for each treatment, and clean and disinfect the handle thoroughly (**11.47**).
- Discharge the air/water syringe without a tip for 20 seconds between each patient; then fit a sterile tip.[4]
- If the dental unit has not been used for some days, discharge the air/water syringe for 2 minutes without the tip.[4] Consider disinfecting the dental unit water supply, if the unit does not have an existing facility.

11.47 Clean and disinfect the handle of the air/water syringe, if it is not autoclavable.

Ultrasonic Scaler

The ultrasonic scaler, and especially its tips, becomes very contaminated during use. Clean and sterilise the ultrasonic scaler after each use. Autoclavable ultrasonic scalers are available (**11.48**).

If it is not possible to sterilise the ultrasonic scaler, the tip must be detached, cleaned, and sterilised after each use (**11.49**). The handle of the scaler should be thoroughly disinfected (**11.50**).

11.48

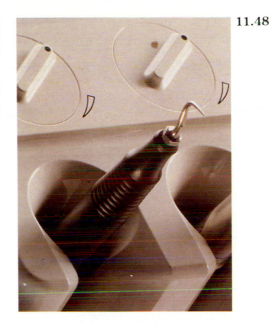

11.48 Autoclavable ultrasonic scaler. (Courtesy Siemens.)

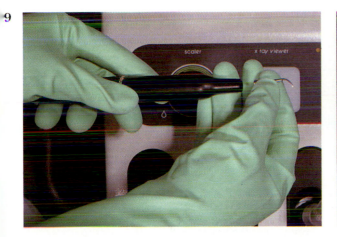

11.49 Detach the autoclavable scaler tip.

11.50

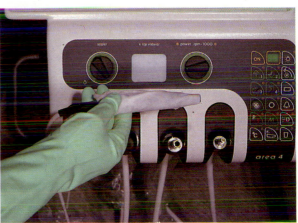

11.50 Wrap the scaler in gauze soaked in iodophore, for 10 minutes.

The Compressor

Install an air-supply system based on a purpose-made dental compressor which will deliver air that is abso-lutely clean and without traces of moisture, particles, oil, or odour.

Checklist

- Install a suitable dental compressor which delivers clean air to the dental unit.
- Choose an oil-free compressor which delivers pure, oil-free air.
- Fit a good-quality dental air filter with an activated charcoal element which will remove airborne impurities and moisture before the air enters the piping network.
- Replace all filter elements regularly, as recommended by the manufacturer.
- Drain the air receiver daily. This removes water which may get into the airline or may become foul.
- Have the compressor serviced regularly.

Servicing dental equipment

The dentist has an obligation to decontaminate any equipment which is to be repaired or serviced by an engineer. Handpieces which are sent for repair must be sterilised if possible.

References

[1]Fitzgibbon, E. J., Bartzokas, C. A., Martin, M. V., Gibson, M. F., Graham, R. The source frequency of bacterial contamination of dental unit water systems. *Br. Dent. J.,* 1984;**157**:98–101.

[2]Bagga, R., Murphy, R., Anderson, A., Punwandi, I. Contamination of dental unit cooling water with oral micro-organisms and its prevention. *J. Am. Dent. Assoc.,* 1984; **109**:712–6.

[3]Mills, S. E., Lauderdale, P. W., Mayhew, R. B. Reduction of microbial contamination in dental units provided with povidone-iodine 10%. *J. Am. Dent. Assoc.,* 1986;**113**: 280–84.

[4]Tippet, B. F., Edwards, J. L., Jenkinson, H. F. Bacterial contamination of dental unit water lines—a possible source of cross infection. *N. Z. Dent. J.,* 1984;**Oct:**112–13.

[5]Crawford, J. J. and Broderius, C. Evaluation of a dental unit designed to prevent retraction of oral fluids. *Quint. Int.,* 1990;**21**:47–51.

[6]Fiehn, N. E. and Henriksen, K. Methods of disinfection of the water system of dental units by water chlorination. *J. Dent. Res.,* 1988;**67**:1499–1504.

[7]Pankhurst, C. C., Philpott–Howard, J., Hewitt, J. H., Casewell, M. W. The efficiency of chlorination and filtration in the control of Legionella from dental chair water systems. *J. Hosp. Inf.,* 1990;**16**:9–18.

[8]Howerton, W. B. and Crawford, J. J. Evaluation and elimination of bacterial contamination in dental unit water systems UNC school of dentistry (unpublished work).

[9]Martin, M. V. The significance of the bacterial contamination of dental unit water systems. *Br. Dent. J.,* 1987;**163**: 152–4.

[10]Gross, A., Devine, M. J., Cutright, G. Microbial contamination of dental units and ultrasonic scalers. *J. Periodont.,* 1976;**47**:670–73.

[11]Murphy, R. A., Boghosian, Kroeger, A. V. Decontamination of dental unit water supplies. *Abstr. Ann. Mtg. Am. Soc. Microbiol.,* 1980;**80**:199.

[12]American Dental Association Council on Dental Materials. Instruments and equipment: dental units and water retraction. *J. Am. Dent. Assoc.,* 1988;**116**:417–20.

[13]Exner, M., Tushewitzki, G., Scharnagel, J. The influence on biofilms by chemical disinfectants and mechanical cleaning. *Zbl. Bact. Hyg.,* 1987;**183**:549–63.

[14]Quincey, E. D., Williams, N. J., Ames, L. L., Ingram, L. R., Covington, J. The air water syringe: contamination and disinfection. *Quint. Int.,* 1989;**20**:911–16.

12. Clinical Waste

USA Regulations

Disposal of infectious waste *within* the dental office is governed by the Occupational Safety and Health Administration (OSHA) regulations. The Environmental Protection Agency (EPA) regulates disposal of infectious waste *after* it has left the dental office.

Despite the OSHA and EPA regulations, dentists continue to be most affected by state and local requirements for handling infectious waste. These regulations and laws vary greatly from state to state. Dentists are advised to check with their state dental association or state environmental protection agency for *specific* state regulations.

There continues to be increasing regulatory activity at both the county and municipality level which may be more restrictive than state regulations. Dentists must be familiar with local government regulations.

Summary of OSHA regulations

For most dental offices only sharps, teeth, and blood-soaked items fit the OSHA definition of infectious waste.

The OSHA rules on waste disposal pertain to safe handling and disposal of such waste while it is in the dental office. OSHA has no jurisdiction over waste *after* it has left the office.

General clinical waste

All infectious waste destined for disposal should be placed in closable, leakproof containers or bags that are colour-coded or labelled. These are placed inside a *second* similar container or bag (closable, leakproof, and colour-coded or labelled) which is closed to prevent leakage during handling, storage, and transport.

Disposal of all infectious waste should be in accordance with applicable federal, state, and local laws.

Sharps

Used needles and other sharps should not be sheared, bent, broken, or re-sheathed by hand. Needles should not be removed from disposable syringes. Mechanical devices or the one-handed scoop technique can be used to re-cap needles.

Immediately after use, sharps should be disposed of in a suitable puncture-resistant container which is labelled or colour-coded. Commercial sharps containers are acceptable. OSHA categorises orthodontic wires as sharps (the EPA does not).

Sharps containers should be located in the immediate area of use and should be easily accessible to personnel, that is, located in each operatory. Sharps containers should not be allowed to overfill.

Labelling

Containers of infectious waste should be either red or labelled. Labels required by OSHA should be of the type illustrated (**12.1**). They should be an integral part of the container.

OSHA regulations state that the employer must establish a training programme for employees relating to disposal of clinical waste.

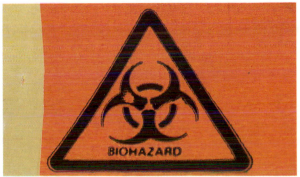

12.1

12.1   A hazard-warning label should be fluorescent orange or orange-red with lettering and symbols in a contrasting colour.

Summary of EPA standards

Tracking and managing waste

The EPA, in response to the Medical Waste Tracking Act (MWTA) of 1988, instituted a two-year demonstration programme governing the handling, tracking, transportation, and disposal of medical waste. It was completed on 22 June 1991. New Jersey, New York, Connecticut, Rhode Island, Louisiana, Washington DC, and Puerto Rico participated in this demonstration programme.

These regulations cover the disposal of sharps, tissue, extracted teeth, and items which are blood-contaminated. Most dental offices will be classed as 'small generators' of infectious waste, i.e. ones which dispose of *less* than 50 lb (22.5 kg) of regulated waste per month.

Larger dental offices may generate more than 50 lb (22.5 kg) of regulated waste a month, and are subjected to more stringent regulations.

The EPA regulations do not overrule state laws, which may be more demanding.

It is likely that the Act will need to be extended for a further two years, to provide Congress with time to adopt a permanent waste statute as part of the existing Resource Conservation Recovery Act.

The main details of EPA standards are summarised below.

Initial packaging—inner container

- Sharps should be placed in a puncture-proof container.
- Blood-soaked items or those caked with blood should be placed in a leak-resistant container.

- Extracted teeth, not returned to a patient or donated to a dental school, should be placed in a sharps container.
- Fluids in volumes of 20 ml or over must be segregated.

Packaging for shipment—outer container

Regulated medical waste must be packaged in outer containers or shipping cartons which:

- Are rigid and leak resistant.
- Are impervious to moisture.
- Will not tear or burst under normal handling conditions.
- Are sealed to prevent leakage when shipping.

If plastic bags are used, they must be red or be marked with a biohazard symbol. The bags must be very strong to prevent tearing, and must be securely sealed.

Labelling of packaging for shipment

Inner container
Red plastic bags or bags having a water-resistant label which includes:

- The words 'medical waste' or 'infectious waste', or the universal biohazard symbol.
- The practitioner's name and address and state permit and identification number (if applicable).

Outer container
A water-resistant tag must be placed on the outer container. The tag must include:

- Generator's or intermediate handler's name and state permit number or identification number (if applicable).
- Transporter's name and address and state permit or identification number (if applicable).
- Date of shipment.
- Identification of contents as medical waste.

Storage of waste on site

Prior to treatment or transport, the generator of waste is required to:

- Maintain the integrity of the packaging and protect it from water, rain, and wind.
- Prevent conditions that will lead to putrification, using refrigeration if necessary.
- Lock outside-storage areas containing medical waste.
- Store waste in a manner that affords protection from animals and insects.

Record keeping

Small generators must maintain logs. Large generators must maintain logs and tracking records. Sample logs and tracking records can be obtained from the American Dental Association (ADA) or EPA.

Shipment of medical waste

Small generators may arrange transport of medical waste in the following ways:

Waste haulers

Practitioners should employ a waste hauler who is registered with the EPA. For more information phone EPA hotline (800) 424-9346. The ADA provides a list of waste haulers, or alternatively contact the state or local dental society and the state environmental agency for information regarding waste haulers. Waste haulers recommended by the ADA are listed in the ADA publication *Infectious Waste Disposal in the Dental Office*, August, 1989.

Choose a waste hauler who complies with local regulations pertaining to infectious waste disposal, and who will indemnify the dentist for its mishandling of infectious waste. Otherwise the dentist is responsible for liability that results from improper disposal of infectious waste by the hauler.

Shipment of sharps

Use a medical waste hauler. Small generators may transport sharps by US registered mail. UPSs are not allowed under EPA regulations. Log requirements apply and should include the name and address of disposal source.

Private vehicles

The small generator may use his or her own vehicle to transport waste to a disposal facility. It is necessary to have a written agreement stipulating that the disposal facility will accept the medical waste. Regulations determining the frequency of disposal vary from state to state.

Destruction on site

Generators of medical waste are exempt from all requirements, except record keeping, if they destroy waste at the site of its generation. The EPA define waste destruction as autoclaving that eliminates the potential of waste to create disease. The requirement for destruction is satisfied when waste is ground or crushed so that it is no longer recognisable.

State regulations

Dentists are advised to check with their state dental association, state environmental protection agency, or state health agency for specific state regulations and should also be aware of local government regulations.

Some important discrepancies between state and EPA regulations exist. For example, some states do not allow 'on site' decontamination, and some states do not have 'small' generator exemptions.

EPA regulations and most state regulations do not include as medical waste, patient disposables such as gloves, drapes, cotton rolls, and gauze unless they are *saturated* with blood. However, some state regulations and proposals include all patient-care disposables as regulated waste (e.g. Pennsylvania and Maryland). It may be safer to treat all patient disposables as medical waste if it is economical and practical, and the resultant increase in weight of all patient disposables does not push the amount of medical waste over 50 lb (22.5 kg) a month.

Inspection of dental offices and penalties

Section 1107(b) of the Resource Conservation and Recovery Act (RCRA) as amended by the MWTA reserves the right of states and localities to adopt and enforce their own laws which may be more stringent than the federal (EPA) regulations.

The EPA is allowing states to take the lead on enforcement and the most likely source of compliance inspection will be the appropriate state agency.

EPA regional officers, if in possession of a warrant, have authority to inspect dental offices. EPA and state penalties can be very severe.

UK Regulations

Health and Safety at Work Act 1974

Section 2(3) of the Act requires that every dental practice has a safety policy which includes instructions on the safe handling, transport, and disposal of clinical waste. Non-compliance with this regulation may result in heavy fines or immediate closure of the dental practice.

Practitioners should be aware that under the Control of Pollution Act (special waste regulations, 1980) they are responsible for the ultimate fate of clinical waste from dental practices.

Department of Health regulations

Regulations are contained in the HMSO publication *Guidance for Clinical Healthcare Workers: Protection Against Infection with HIV and Hepatitis Viruses*.

Section 2.4.4 (p. 21) describes disposal of clinical waste excluding sharps; advising disposal in accordance with the HSAS document *The Safe Disposal of Clinical Waste*, HMSO, 1982, ISBN 0 11 88364112.

Section 2.4.5 describes disposal of sharps; advising disposal in accordance with the publication *Used Sharps Disposal*, SIB (87) 31 March, 1987. Dentists are advised to purchase sharps containers complying with the new British Standard BS7320:1990.

Practitioners in the UK must be familiar with these regulations, and those working under the National Health regulations who do not comply may be found 'in breach of terms of service'.

General Dental Council

The General Dental Council in its latest *Notice for the Guidance of Dentists* states under Paragraph 17 'a dentist has a duty to take appropriate precautions to protect his staff and his patients from the risk of cross infection in the dental surgery. Failure to provide and use adequate sterilization facilities may render a dentist liable to proceedings for misconduct.' (This may include failure to dispose of contaminated clinical waste safely.)

Environmental Protection Act 1990

This Act covers the disposal of sharps and medical waste and mandates that dentists must use a medical waste contractor who is registered with a waste control authority.

Disposal of Clinical Waste and Sharps

Disposable sharp objects

Used anaesthetic needles, disposable scalpels, anaesthetic cartridges, used burs, orthodontic wire, extracted teeth, and other sharp objects should be carefully dropped into a solid puncture-resistant container (**12.2 & 12.3**). Such containers should be labelled according to relevant local environmental regulations. They are filled no more than two-thirds full and then sealed. Sharps containers should be incinerated.

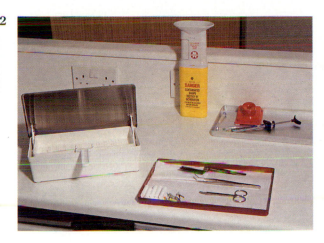

12.2   The sharps container may be located near to the operating zone.

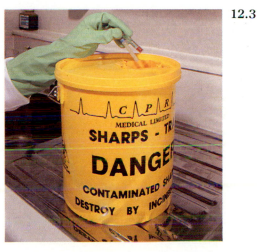

12.3   Larger containers located in sterilisation area.

Contaminated solid medical waste

Materials that are soaked in blood, e.g. blood contaminated gauze, cotton rolls, gowns, patient bibs, masks, gloves, and other soft items should be carefully placed into a waste receiver containing a *strong* bin liner. Care should be taken to avoid contamination of areas around the waste receiver or the outer surface of the bin liner (**12.4**). Bin liners with side handles facilitate safe removal and tying.

When the bin liner is two-thirds full it should be removed from the waste receiver and sealed or tied (**12.5**). Waste should not remain in the waste receiver overnight. It has been suggested that waste

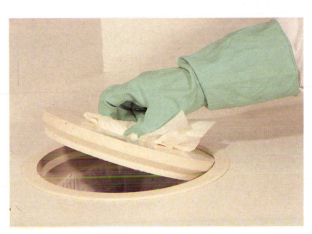

12.4   The lid of the waste receiver is removed using a tissue.

155

receivers should be emptied and new bin liners fitted, before treating a medically compromised patient.

The bin liner should then be carefully placed into a strong plastic red (USA) or yellow (UK) bag (**12.6**) which should be clearly marked according to relevant regulations. These bags should be sealed and later incinerated. Take care not to contaminate the outer surface of the second bag.

When handling clinical waste, wear heavy-duty utility gloves.

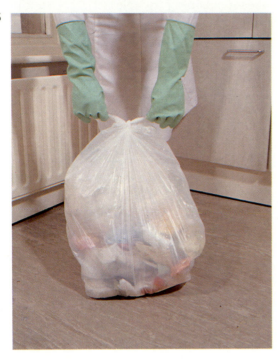

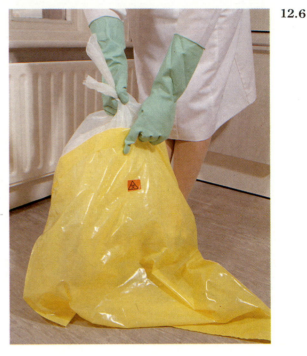

12.5   Seal the bin liner when two-thirds full.

12.6   The outer bag. The label on this bag does not meet OSHA regulations as it cannot be clearly identified at a distance of 5 feet (1.5 metres).

Liquid waste

Liquid waste includes bulk blood and suctioned or waste-trap fluids. Small quantities of these liquids may be poured into a drain or toilet that is connected to a sanitary sewer system. Wear heavy utility gloves, protective goggles, and a mask.

All liquid waste and contaminated medical waste should be disposed of according to national or local environmental regulations.

Storage

Store medical waste bags and sharps containers in locked safe areas according to local regulations.

Transportation of contaminated waste and sharps

In the UK, each Family Health Authority organises weekly medical waste and sharps collections from dental offices. This waste is then incinerated.

Collection and transportation of sharps and clinical waste in the USA should be carried out according to federal state or local laws and regulations.

13. Prosthetics and Orthodontics

Prosthetics

Risks

There is limited evidence of transmission of infection to the dental technician through direct contact with contaminated impressions and prostheses.[1,2] Dental prostheses and impressions may prove a hazard to the dentist and dental assistant who handle them after removal from the mouth.

A study[3] has found that 67% of materials sent from dental offices to laboratories were contaminated with bacteria of varying degrees of pathogenicity. With care this risk can be substantially reduced.

Good cross infection control is essential both in the dental office and in the dental laboratory.

Cross infection control in the dental office

Practitioners should implement cross infection control described in American Dental Association (ADA) and Centers for Disease Control (CDC) guidelines. Follow the principles described with regard to critical, semi-critical, and non-critical instruments whenever possible.

Many items and instruments used in prosthetics cannot be heat sterilised nor subjected to prolonged high-level disinfection without damage. The majority do not have direct contact with blood and oral fluid and may be considered non-critical. Some have direct contact with blood and are classed as semi-critical.

Semi-critical instruments and items

The following instruments and items should be subjected to heat sterilisation or high-level disinfection. If damage occurs with prolonged high-level disinfection, compromise medium-level disinfection with a tuberculocidal hospital infectant is recommended.

- Impressions: medium-level disinfection.
- Prostheses which have been worn and are either adjusted in the surgery, or repaired or adjusted in the laboratory: medium-level disinfection.
- The face bow fork: heat sterilisation.
- Wax knife, if used for adjustments at the chairside: heat sterilisation.
- Prostheses, at try-in stage: medium-level disinfection.
- Metal dispensing syringes for impressions should be cleaned and heat sterilised.
- Bite blocks: medium-level disinfection
- Polishing stones and rag wheels: heat-sterilisation if possible.
- Impression trays returned from the laboratory: aluminium or chrome plated—heat sterilisation, plastic—discard.
- The handles of disposable trays can be detached and autoclaved but corrosion and rusting may occur after a few cycles. Sterilisation using a chemiclave may be preferred.

Non-critical instruments

These non-critical items should be disinfected with a medium-level tuberculocidal hospital disinfectant using the spray–wipe–spray technique.

- Articulators and face bows (without the face and bow fork).
- Mixing bowls and spatulas. (Some stainless-steel mixing bowls and autoclavable spatulas are available. These may be heat sterilised if preferred.)
- Shade and mold guides—if the shade guides are disinfected using an iodophor, wipe immediately with alcohol or water to avoid discoloration.[4]
- Prosthetic rulers.
- Wax rims should be discarded.

Unit-dose concept

This means dispensing, prior to patient contact, a sufficient amount of a material needed to accomplish a procedure. Any excess is discarded on completion.[5]

The unit-dose concept minimises the chances of cross infection during prosthetic procedures.[4] To minimise contamination of packaged items stored in drawers or cupboards, unit doses of impression materials, wax, etc. should be dispensed before beginning the procedure. *See* Chapter 7.

Bite blocks and prostheses at the try-in stage

These should be disinfected by immersion in a medium-level tuberculocidal hospital disinfectant for the recommended time.

- Disinfect bite blocks and 'try-ins' which have been returned from the laboratory, *before* fitting.
- Disinfect bite blocks and 'try-ins' after fitting, before they are returned to the laboratory.

Procedure

Immersion in sodium hypochlorite: bleach (5.25% sodium hypochlorite) is diluted 1:10, i.e. 1 part bleach to 9 parts water. Immersion time is 10 minutes (**13.1 & 13.2**).

Decontamination should be carried out in the **dental surgery**, not in the dental laboratory or in both.

A package sticker or instructions on the work sheet should inform the dental technician that these items have been disinfected.

13.1

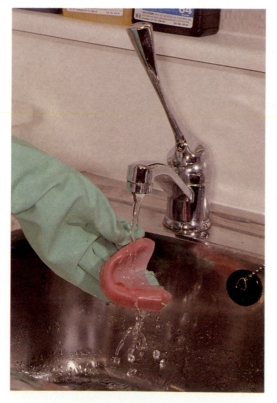

13.1 Thoroughly rinse the item under tap water.

13

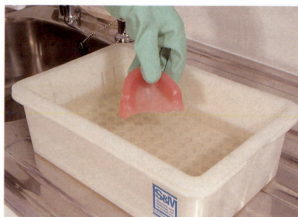

13.2 Disinfect for 10 minutes, then thoroughly rinse under tap water to remove residual disinfectant.

Impressions

Impressions have been shown to be contaminated on arrival at dental laboratories[3] and casts poured in non-disinfected impressions have been shown to contain micro-organisms.[6] ADA guidelines state the impressions 'should be rinsed to remove saliva, blood, and debris and then disinfected' before being sent to the laboratory.

Stability of impression materials following disinfection of materials is a major concern, and it has been established that distortion of impressions may occur following some disinfection routines.

Some impression materials used in dentistry

- **Condensation silicones/polysulphide materials**
  (condensation reaction polysiloxane)

  Products
  Optosil
  Permalistic
  Deguflex
  Xantopren
  Coltex, medium, fine, extra fine
  Zetaplus
  Coltoflax
  Rapid

- **Addition cured silicones**
  (vinyl polysiloxane)

  Products
  Reprosil
  Express
  President
  Elite
  Provil
  Panasil
  Basilex
  Imprint
  Extrude
  Unosil S

- **Polyether impressions**

  Products
  Impregnum F
  Permadyne

- **Alginate**
  (irreversible hydrocolloids)

  Products
  Alginoplast
  New Kromopan
  Jeltrate
  Xantalgin
  Blueprint Cremix, Rapid and Asept
  SS White DSA
  CA 37
  Zelgan

- **Agar**
  (reversible hydrocolloids)

  Products
  VAR R Heavybody

- **Zinc Oxide Eugenol (ZOE)**
  (impression paste)

  Products
  SS White impression paste
  Cavex

- **Compound**

  Products
  Kerr green compound
  Kerr red compound

Disinfection of impressions

- Immersion disinfection has been preferred to spraying. This is based on the assumption that immersion is more likely to assure exposure of *all* surfaces of the impression to the disinfectant for the recommended time.[5]
- Spraying disinfectants onto the surface of the impression reduces the chance of distortion, especially in the case of alginate, hydrocolloid, and polyether materials, but may not adequately cover areas of undercut. Two studies have indicated that there is no difference in accuracy of casts obtained by spraying with or immersion in recommended disinfectants.[7,8]
- Thorough rinsing of the impression is necessary *before and after* disinfection. Rinsing before re- moves the bioburden present, which may prevent exposure of the surface to the disinfectant. Rinsing after disinfection removes residual disinfectant which may affect the stone surface after casting.[5]
- ADA recommended disinfectants must be used:[5]
    chlorine compounds
    iodophors
    combination synthetic phenolics
    glutaraldehydes.
- Distortion of impressions following disinfection is determined by the brand of impression material and the disinfectant used.[7,9,10]

When an alginate is disinfected the choice of product is *very* important.[7]

Polysulphides and addition-cured silicones

Addition-cured silicones and polysulphide impressions have been shown to be generally stable when immersed in ADA recommended tuberculocidal hospital disinfectants.[10–15]

The recommended procedure for disinfection is shown in **13.3 & 13.4**.

Note: Addition-cured silicone materials appear to be able to withstand damage by disinfectants, with the exception of neutral glutaraldehyde.[10]

Alternative disinfectant: iodophore.

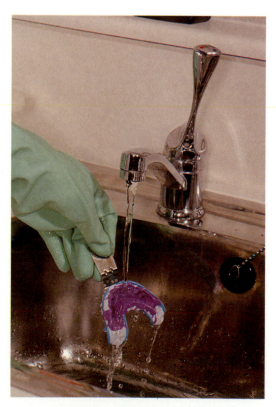

13.3 Thoroughly rinse the impression under running tap water. Avoid excessive splashing.

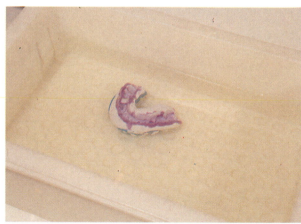

13.4 Immerse the impression in sodium hypochlorite (dilute 1 part bleach with 9 parts water) for 10 minutes. Rinse the impression thoroughly under running tap water to remove residual traces of disinfectant. Shake to remove residual water.

Alginate

Alginate is a complete carbohydrate that imbibes water. Immersion disinfection for long periods will cause a distortion of alginate impressions due to the intake of water and the action of the disinfectant. Avoid prolonged immersion.

Investigations to evaluate the stability of alginate impressions following disinfection, have produced varying results, depending on the techniques and materials evaluated.[9,13,16–18]

Recommended procedure

- Rinse the impression thoroughly under running tap water, shake the impression to remove excess water.
- Dip the impression in a 1:10 solution of sodium hypochlorite for several seconds to ensure maximum contact of undercut with the disinfectant (**13.5**).
- Wrap the impression in gauze soaked in 1:10 sodium hypochlorite, place in a plastic bag and seal for 10 minutes (**13.6**).
- Remove the impression and rinse thoroughly under running tap water.

Recent research has indicated that inactivation of viruses may be highly unpredictable when a disinfectant is sprayed onto impressions. Simple spray disinfection and an immediate rinse should not in general be considered an appropriate method.[19]

Immersion of alginate

Immersion of alginates in disinfectants is very much dependant on the product used.

Algioplast and **New Kromopan** may be immersed in sodium hypochlorite solution (1:10) for 10 minutes without distortion.[20]

Jeltrate Plus may be immersed in iodophor (wescodyne) for 10–15 minutes[21], or for 10 minutes in sodium hypochlorite[22], without distortion.

It is strongly recommended that alginate impressions are cast as soon as possible after disinfection. This is possible if the dental office has its own laboratory, but difficult if commercial laboratories are employed.

Alginate impregnated with disinfectant

Disinfectants such as didecyl-dimethyl ammonium chloride have been impregnated into alginate. One such product is commercially available (Blueprint Asept).

A recent study[23] recommended Blueprint Asept as an effective means of reducing the number of viable micro-organisms surviving on the actual impression, but the problem of microbial contamination of the impression tray itself remains.

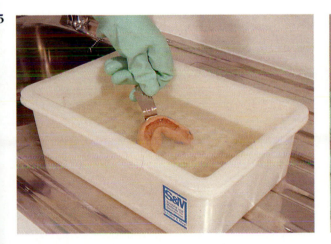

13.5 Disinfection of alginate with sodium hypochlorite.

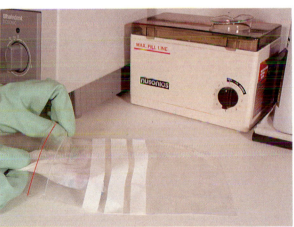

13.6 Place the impression, wrapped in soaked gauze, in a plastic bag.

Polyether impressions

Research results with polyether impressions have also varied.[10,13,14,24] Care must be taken, as some distortion is possible after prolonged immersion. Sodium hypochlorite 1:10 should be used.

- Rinse the impression thoroughly, shake off excess water.
- Dip the impression in sodium hypochlorite solution for several seconds and remove.
- Wrap the impression in gauze soaked with sodium hypochlorite and place the impression in a sealed bag for 10 minutes.
- Remove the impression from the bag and rinse.

Note: Polyether impressions (Impregnum) have been found to stand immersion for 10 minutes in a disinfectant (Gigasept, Sterling Medicare UK) without distortion. Short immersion times are recommended.[25] A further study indicates that immersion of polyether impressions for short periods may be acceptable.[26]

Agar—reversible hydrocolloids

Reversible hydrocolloids have been shown to be stable when immersed in 1:10 sodium hypochlorite or 1:213 iodophor.[21,27,28]

Recommendation
Immerse in sodium hypochlorite solution (1:10) for 10 minutes using the procedure described for addition-cured silicone materials.

Alternative disinfectant—iodophor
It has been found that immersion in iodophor solution (Wescodyne) is a safe and effective method for disinfecting agar materials.[21]

Zinc oxide eugenol (ZOE) and compound impressions

Only limited data are available on the disinfection of zinc oxide eugenol[30,31] and compound impressions.[32]

Zinc oxide eugenol
Immersion in 2% glutaraldehyde or a 1:213 iodophore solution for 10 minutes.[31] Materials disinfected with glutaraldehyde should be thoroughly rinsed to remove residual traces of the disinfectant. Glutaraldehyde is a strong irritant to the skin and mucous membranes.

Compound
Immersion in sodium hypochlorite (bleach, diluted 1:10).[5,32]

Impression trays

If plastic disposable trays are used, the handle is removed and heat sterilised.

If aluminium or chrome-plated trays are used, routine examination of the trays is essential to monitor corrosion if sodium hypochlorite is used. If corrosion occurs, use an alternative disinfectant.

Disinfecting prostheses

Disinfect prostheses and appliances before returning them to a dental laboratory, following insertion into the mouth.

Disinfect prostheses and appliances returned from a dental laboratory, before insertion into the mouth. The procedure is illustrated (**13.7 & 13.8**).

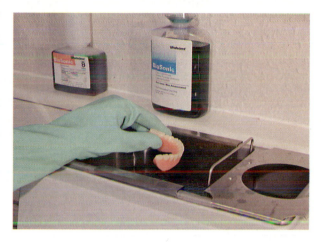

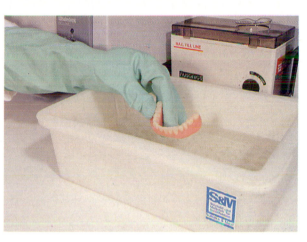

13.7 Clean the prostheses for 6 minutes in an ultrasonic cleaner. Use an all-purpose, mild, detergent ultrasonic cleaning fluid. Rinse the prostheses under tap water. Shake the appliance to remove excess water.

13.8 Disinfect the prostheses for 10 minutes in sodium hypochlorite (1:10). Rinse the prostheses under tap water thoroughly. Alternative disinfectant—iodophor.

Choice of disinfectant

Metal dentures

Some concern has been expressed over the use of dilute sodium hypochlorite on metal dentures. Recent research[33,34] indicates that the use of sodium hypochlorite for 10 minutes will not damage denture base metals. One study recommends 2% hypochlorite 1:5 for 5 minutes, as 1% does not remove all microorganisms.[28]

Other studies conclude that sodium hypochlorite should not be used and that iodophors are the first choice disinfectants.[5,35]

Iodophor or 1:10 diluted sodium hypochlorite may be used for single or infrequent disinfection cycles. However, both disinfectants should be used with care as either can be corrosive with repeated or prolonged exposure.

Acrylic dentures

Sodium hypochlorite is recommended for disinfection of complete acrylic dentures.[36,37] Glutaraldehyde with phenolic buffer (Sporacidin) should not be used.[38]

'In-office' adjustments

Care must be taken with in-office adjustments. Use sterilised rag wheels and unit doses of pumice and polishing compounds. These will prevent cross contamination of prostheses and the need for multiple disinfections when repeat try-ins are necessary.[5]

Changing disinfectant solutions

Disinfectant solutions recommended should be changed *daily*.

Manufacturer's recommendations

Refer to the manufacturer's recommendations before undertaking any of the procedures described.

Note: A recent study[39] indicated that some impression manufacturers do not have appropriate complete disinfection protocols.

Cross infection control in the dental laboratory

Communication with dental laboratory staff

Responsibility for disinfection of items sent to the dental laboratory lies with the dental office.[40] All items disinfected in the dental office should be labelled, indicating that such items have been decontaminated using an accepted disinfection routine. This will avoid duplicating disinfection procedures which may damage materials.

Materials returned to the dentist from a laboratory should be disinfected in the dental office prior to fitting.

Mutual communication of infection control routines in the office and the laboratory is *essential* to prevent duplication of such routines.

'In-house' dental laboratories

Infection control routines are easily delegated be-tween the dental office and the laboratory.

Commercial dental laboratories

Many items received from dental offices are con-taminated.[3] This leads to the assumption that most items arriving at the dental laboratory have not been disinfected.

The majority of the routines described below are unnecessary if good cross infection control is pract-ised by the dental office and communicated to the dental laboratory. However, unless laboratory staff are certain that this is the case, cross infection control procedures should be undertaken at the laboratory to protect staff.

Cross infection control routines

Receiving area

All items received from dental offices are placed in this area. The items are unpacked by a member of the laboratory staff wearing heavy rubber utility gloves, a mask, and protective eyewear. The packaging is disposed of as contaminated medical waste.

If the dental laboratory staff have not been notified that incoming work is decontaminated, all incoming items must be disinfected using routines described in this section. Boxes for work should be disinfected after unloading.

Receiving area benches are thoroughly disinfected after dealing with each case, using a recommended hard-surface disinfectant.

Casting impressions

If impressions are carefully disinfected, precautions to prevent contamination of stone models are unneces-sary.

As an alternative to disinfecting impressions, other techniques have been suggested:

- Stone models may be sprayed with an iodophor or with sodium hypochlorite prior to handling,[41,42] or the dental cast may be soaked for one hour in 5.25% sodium hypochlorite saturated with dental stone (calcium sulphate dihydrate).
- Disinfectant may be added to the gauging liquid. A recent study suggests that sterilisation of a cast poured against a contaminated impression is pos-sible by adding 25% by volume of commercial bleach to the gauging liquid without affecting cast accuracy, hardness, or surface character.

The set of a cast can be accelerated to be compatible with hydrocolloid impression materials by adding 50% slurry when making up the gauging liquid. Mix 25% water, 25% sodium hypochlorite, and 50% slurry as a gauging liquid. A biologically safe cast can be produced from contaminated impressions.[22]

Microwaves are unacceptable for sterilising dental casts.[22,43]

Polishing prostheses

Studies have described contamination of pumice and polishing lathes[44], contaminated aerosol following polishing[45] and transmission of infection to a technician.[46]

Add 3 parts of green soap to the disinfectant solution (5 parts sodium hypochlorite to 100 parts distilled water) before mixing the pumice. This helps to keep the pumice suspended. The pumice should be changed daily and the lathe disinfected. Unit doses of pumice may be used in each case and then discarded. The technician should wear protective eyewear and a mask when polishing. Polishing lathes are available with integral dust-chip evacuators (**13.9**). Use a new sterile rag wheel when polishing a prosthetic appliance.

Special precautions when handling used prostheses

Acrylic prostheses that have been worn for some time are porous; grinding of the surface may expose micro-organisms that have not been subjected to disinfection procedures. It has been suggested that gloves should be worn when grinding 'old' acrylic, despite the danger of gloves becoming caught up in polishing instruments. The US National Association of Dental Laboratories does not suggest the use of gloves for grinding disinfected prostheses, it suggests having a disinfectant at the lathe side for immediate disinfection following exposure by grinding of previously worn prostheses.

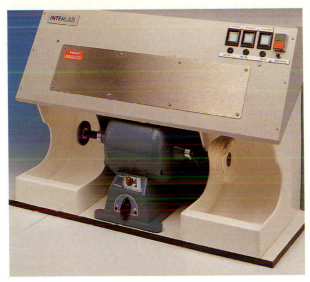

13.9 Polishing lathe.

Other precautions

- Technicians should be vaccinated against infectious diseases, e.g. hepatitis B.
- Frequent hand washing is essential.
- Work gowns should be changed frequently.
- Work benches, sinks, and equipment in the production area should be cleaned and disinfected daily.
- Do not eat in the laboratory.
- Sterilise burs and stones.
- Instruments, attachments, and materials used with new prostheses and other appliances should be separate from those used on prostheses and appliances which have previously been inserted in the mouth.
- Disinfect bristle brushes and rinse with water.
- Discard impression material from the tray and the bite registration wax.
- Outgoing cases should be disinfected before they are returned to the dental office unless the dental office staff undertake disinfection procedures.

Orthodontics

Orthodontists have the second highest incidence of hepatitis B among dental professionals.[47]

Orthodontic procedures include banding, bonding, re-tries, arch wire changes, delivery of removable appliances, and band removal. A recent survey indicates that an orthodontist or chairside assistant receives an average of about one cut per week.[48]

The process of cleaning and sterilising orthodontic instruments presents special problems. These instruments have large hinge areas that are difficult to clean and sterilise. They also have sharp angles, cutting edges, and pointed ends that are easily damaged.

Orthodontic instruments, especially orthodontic pliers, may be damaged after repeated autoclave cycles, although one study has suggested that pliers may be autoclaved without damage.[49] Chrome-plated pliers are more resistant to damage during autoclaving than stainless-steel pliers.[49] Lubrication of the hinges should be carried out prior to autoclaving, and the pliers should be dipped in 1.0% sodium nitrate before autoclaving.

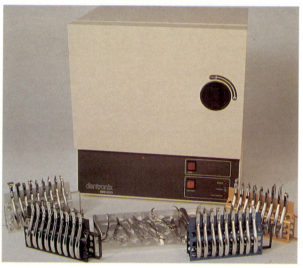

13.10 The DDS 5000 steriliser.

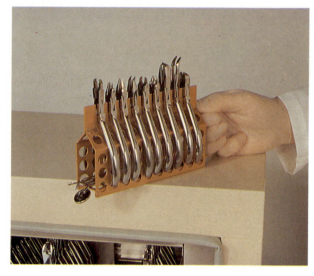

13.11 The orthodontic plier rack.

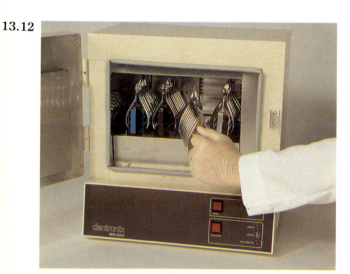

13.12 The DDS 5000 fully loaded.

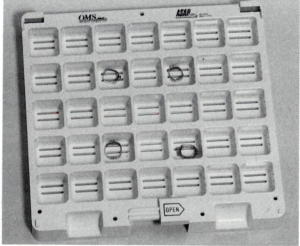

13.13 Band cassette with stainless-steel orthodontic bands and brackets. (Courtesy Drs W. Hohlt, C. Miller, J. Neeb, M. Sheldrake, and the *American Journal of Orthodontics and Dentofacial Orthopedics.*)

The chemical vapour steriliser has been used to sterilise orthodontic instruments and there is minimal corrosion and damage to cutting edges when using this type of steriliser.

Convection heat has become a popular means of sterilisation of instruments for orthodontic offices. The Cox rapid heat steriliser and the Dentronix DDS 5000 are becoming widely used and both sterilisers have rapid cycles.

The Cox steriliser has three optional cycles which vary in time according to the items to be sterilised. The 6-minute cycle is used for unwrapped instruments; and packaged instruments undergo a 12-minute cycle. Approximately 25 orthodontic pliers fit comfortably on the removable tray. A fan cools the instruments after the completion of the cycle, and orthodontic pliers are cool enough to use 10 minutes after the cycle is completed. The total sterilisation time required to produce a supply of cool orthodontic instruments is 16 minutes.[50]

The DDS 5000 dry-heat steriliser (**13.10**) is supplied with racks that hold 9 pliers in an upright position (**13.11**) and several more placed horizontally inside the racks. The racks should not be overloaded. Four racks fit into the steriliser chamber (**13.12**), making it possible to sterilise 36 orthodontic pliers in one cycle. Instruments are cool to the touch shortly after the sterilisation cycle is completed, because of an internal fan. The entire sterilisation cycle lasts approximately 22 minutes,[50] which includes warm up (9 minutes), sterilisation (6 minutes) and cool down (7 minutes). Loaded instrument racks are ultrasonically cleaned for 12 minutes prior to sterilisation.

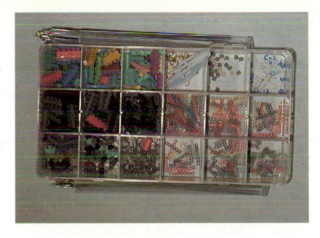

13.14 Unused chain and elastomeric ligatures in a tackle box. (Courtesy Dr M.A. Baron.)

Care should be taken when ultrasonically cleaning pin and ligature cutters as disruption of the insert brazing may occur.[51]

Contaminated bands, arch wires, and brackets may be sterilised in band cassettes (**13.13**) using rapid dry heat, steam or chemical vapour sterilisation.[52]

Alternatively, bands and arch wires may be immersed in 2% glutaraldehyde overnight. Residual traces of glutaraldehyde should be rinsed away.

Unused chain and elastomeric ligatures may be safely stored in a tackle box until they are required. They may be removed with sterilised tweezers (**13.14**).

References

[1]Sabatini, B. M. Don't let it happen to you. Precautions against Hepatitis B and other infectious diseases. *J. Mich. Dent. Assoc.*, 1985;**67**:72–3.

[2]Polayes, I. M. and Arons, M. S. The treatment of Herpetic Whitlow. *Plast. Recon. Surg.*, 1980;**65**:811–17.

[3]Powell, E. L., Runnells, R. D., Saxon, B. A., Whisenani, B. K. The presence and identification of organisms transmitted to dental laboratories. *J. Prosthet. Dent.*, 1990;**64**:235–7.

[4]Stern, M. A. and Whitacre, R. J. Avoiding cross contamination in prosthodontics. *J. Prosthet. Dent.*, 1981;**46**:120–22.

[5]Merchant, V. A. and Molinari, J. Infection control in prosthetics; a choice no longer. *Gen. Dent.*, 1989;**37(1)**:23–32.

[6]Leung, R. L. and Schonfeld, S. E. Gypsum casts as a potential source of microbial contamination. *J. Prosthet. Dent.*, 1983;**49**:210–11.

[7]Matyas, A. S. D., Dao, A. A., Caputo, A. A., Lucatorto, F. M. Effects of disinfectants on dimensional accuracy of impression materials. *J. Prosthet. Dent.*, 1990;**64**:25–31.

[8]Drennon, D., Johnson, G., Powell, L. The accuracy of and efficacy of disinfection by spray atomization on elastomeric impressions. *J. Prosthet. Dent.*, 1989;**62**:468–75.

[9]Peutzfeldt, A. and Asmussen, E. Effect of disinfecting solutions on accuracy of alginate and elastomeric impression materials. *Scand. J. Dent. Res.*, 1989;**97**:470–75.

[10]Johnson, G. A. and Drennon, D. G. Accuracy of elastomeric impressions by immersion. *J. Am. Dent. Assoc.*, 1988;**116**:523–30.

[11]Herrera, S. P. and Merchant, V. A. Dimensional stability of dental impressions after immersion disinfection. *J. Am. Dent. Assoc.*, 1986;**113**:419–22.

[12]Bergman, M., Olsson, S., Bergman, B. Elastomeric impression material: Dimensional stability and surface detail sharpness following treatment with disinfection solutions. *Swed. Dent. J.*, 1980;**4**:161–7.

[13]Herrera, S. P. and Stackhouse, J. A. Dimensional stability of dental impressions after immersion disinfection and cold sterilization. *J. Am. Dent. Assoc.*, 1986;**113**:419–22.

[14]Johansen, R. E. and Stackhouse, J. A. Dimensional changes of elastomers during cold sterilization. *J. Prosthet. Dent.*, 1987;**57**:233–6.

[15]Merchant, V. A., Herrera, S. P., Dwan, J. J. Marginal fit from disinfected elastomeric impressions. *J. Prosthet. Dent.*, 1987;**58**:276–80.

[16]Setcos, J. C., Penj, L., Palenik, C. J. The effect of disinfection procedures on an alginate impression material. *J. Dent. Res.* (Abstract), 1984;**63**:235–6.

[17]Bergman, B., Bergman, M., Olsson, S. Alginate impression materials, dimensional stability and surface detail sharpness following treatment with disinfectant solutions. *Swed. Dent. J.*, 1985;**9**:255–62.

[18]Durr, D. P. and Novak, E. V. Dimensional stability of alginate impressions immersed in disinfecting solutions. *ASDC. J. Dent. Child.*, 1987;**54**:45–8.

[19]Look, J. O., Clay, D. J., Gong, K., Messer, H. H. Preliminary results from disinfection of irreversible hydrocolloid impressions. *J. Prosthet. Dent.*, 1990;**63**:701–7.

[20]Wilson, S. J. and Wilson, H. J. The effect of chlorinated disinfecting solutions on alginate impression materials. *Restor. Dent.*, 1987;**3**:86–9.

[21]Giblin, J., Podesta, R., White, J. Dimensional stability of impression materials immersed in an iodophor disinfectant. *Int. J. Prosthodont.*, 1990;**3**:72–7.

[22]Engelmeier, R. C., Tebrock, O. C., Mayfiel, T. G., Adams, H. J. U. Multiple barrier system. *J. Calif. Dent. Assoc.*, 1988;**16(12)**:17–22.

[23]Ghani, F., Hobkirk, J. A., Wilson, M. Evaluation of a new antiseptic containing alginate impression material. *Br. Dent. J.*, 1990;**169**:83–6.

[24]Setcos, J. C., Gerstenblath, R., Panenik, C. J., Hinoura, K. Disinfection of a polyether dental impression material. *J. Dent. Res.* (Abstract), 1985;**64**:244–5.

[25]McCormick, R. J., Watts, D. C., Wilson, N. H. F. Effects of a solution of succinic aldehyde on elastomeric impressions. *J. Dent.*, 1989;**17**:246–9.

[26]Tullner, J. B., Commette, J. A., Moon, P. C. Linear dimensional changes in dental materials after immersion in a disinfectant solution. *J. Prosthet. Dent.*, 1988;**60**:725–8.

[27]Minagi, S., Yano, N., Yoshida, K., Tsuru, H. Prevention of acquired immunodeficiency syndrome and hepatitis B: disinfection method for hydrophilic impression materials. *J. Prosthet. Dent.*, 1987;**58**:462–5.

[28]Townsend, J. D., Nicholls, J. I., Powell, G. L. The effect of disinfectants on the accuracy of hydrocolloid impression materials. *J. Dent. Res.* (Abstract No. 202), 1988;**67**:138.

[29]Storer, R. and McCabe, J. F. An investigation of methods available for sterilizing impressions. *Br. Dent. J.*, 1981; **151**: 217–19.

[30]Olsson, S., Bergmann, B., Bergman, M. Zinc oxide—eugenol impression materials. Dimensional stability and surface detail sharpness following treatment with disinfectant solutions. *Scand. Dent. J.*, 1982;**6**:177–80.

[31]Merchant, V. A., Stone, C. R., Badr, S. E., Gleason, M. J. Dimensional stability of disinfected zinc oxide eugenol impressions. *J. Dent.Res.*, 1990;**69**(S):304.

[32]Stone, C. R., Badr. S. E., Gleason, M. J., Merchant, V. A. Dimensional stability of disinfected compound impressions. *J. Dent. Res.*, 1989;**68**(S):398.

[33]Casper, R. L., Eric, J. D., Moore, D. J. Corrosion of chrome cobalt alloy by various disinfectants. *J. Dent. Res.*, 1988;**67**:135–6.

[34]McGowan, M. J., Shimoda, L. M., Woolsey, G. D. Effects of sodium hypochlorite on dental base metals during immersion for short-term sterilization. *J. Prosthet. Dent.*, 1988; **60**:212–18.

[35]Merchant, V. A. Disinfection of dental impressions and prostheses. Oakland Co. (Michigan) *Dental Rev.*, 1986; **26**: 14–18, 29.

[36]Rudd, R. W., Senia, E. S., McCleskey, F. K., Adams, E. D. Sterilization of complete dentures with sodium hypochlorite. *J. Prosthetic. Dent.*, 1984;**51**:318–21.

[37]Bell, J. A., Brockman, M. S., Feil, E. D., Sackuvich, D. A. The effectiveness of two disinfectants on dental base acrylic resin with organic load. *J. Prosthet. Dent.*, 1989; **61**: 500–503.

[38]Shen, C., Javid, N. S., Colaizzi, F. A. The effect of glutaraldehyde on dental base resins. *J. Prosthet. Dent.*, 1989;**61**:583–9.

[39]Cottone, J. A., Young, J., Parvin, D. Disinfection/sterilization protocols recommended by manufacturers of impression materials. *Int. J. Prothodont.*, 1990;**3**:379–83.

[40]DLICC Guidelines. *DLICC Infection Control Procedures.* Boston Dental Laboratory Infection Control Council, 1986.

[41]Shaefer, M. E. Infection control in dental laboratory procedures. *Can. Dent. Assoc. J.*, 1985;**13**:81–4.

[42]Sarma, A. C. and Neiman, R. A study of disinfectant chemicals on the physical properties of die stone. *Quint. Int.*, 1990:**21**:53–9.

[43]Davis, D. R., Curtis, D. A., White, J. M. Microwave irradiation of contaminated dental casts. *Quint. Int.*, 1989; **20**:583–5.

[44]Kahn, R. C., Lancaster, M. V., Kate, W. The microbiological cross contamination of dental prostheses. *J. Prosthet. Dent.*, 1982;**47**:556–9.

[45]Miller, R. L., Burton, W. E., Spose, W. E. Aerosols produced by dental instrumentation. *Proc. First Int. Symp. Aerobiol.*, Berkeley California, 1963.

[46]Savide, M. A., Gadof, F., Wenzel, P. P. Point source epidemic of mycoplasma pneumonia infection in a prosthodontics laboratory. *Am. Rev. Respir. Dis.* 1975;**112**:213–17.

[47]Starnbach, H. and Biddle, P. A pragmatic approach to asepsis in the orthodontic office. *Angle Orthod.*, 1988;**50**:63–6.

[48]Cash, R. G. Trends in the sterilization and disinfection procedures in orthodontic offices. *Am. J. Orth. Dentofac. Ortho.*, 1990;**98**:292–9.

[49]Jones, M. L. An initial assessment of the effect on orthodontic pliers of various sterilization disinfection regimes. *Br. J. Orthod.*, 1989;**16**:251–8.

[50]Johnson, M. W., Moore, W. C., Rodu, B. Comparison of convection and heat sterilization units for the orthodontic office. *Am. J. Orthod. Dentofac. Orthop.*, 1991;**99**:57–63.

[51]Murick, J. F. Upgrading sterilization in orthodontic practice. *Am. J. Orthod.*, 1986;**89**:346–51.

[52]Hohlt, W. F., Miller, C. H., Neeb, J. M., Sheldrake, M. A. Sterilization of orthodontic instruments in bands and cassettes. *Am. J. Orthod. Dentofac. Orthop.*, 1990;**98**: 411–16.

14. Infection Control in Endodontics

It is essential to clean and sterilise all instruments used within the root canal thoroughly; the risk of cross infection is very high, if contaminated instruments are used to perform endodontic techniques.

Stage One: Precleaning disinfection

Endodontic files and drills are placed into a holding solution after use (**14.1**). Plastic handles on some endodontic files may be damaged by synthetic phenolic disinfectants; use instruments with metal handles to overcome this problem.

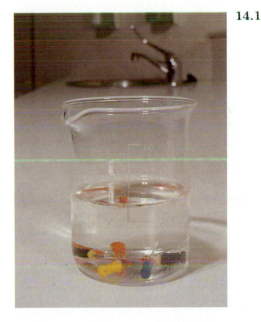

14.1

14.1 A small beaker containing holding solution.

Stage Two: Ultrasonic cleaning

Ultrasonic cleaning may be achieved using a small beaker suspended in the ultrasonic bath (**14.2**). It is important to check files and drills for residual debris; this *must* be removed.

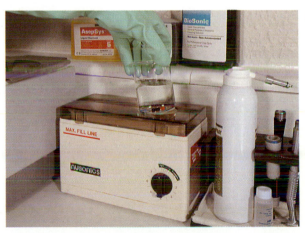

14.2

14.2 Ultrasonic cleaning of endodontic files and drills.

Stage Three: Sterilisation

Endodontic instrument trays or containers should be used (**14.3 & 14.4**). These allow a well organised approach to the sterilisation of endodontic instruments and facilitate safe aseptic storage.

Heat sterilisation, using the chemiclave or the autoclave, will not damage endodontic files[1] and stainless steel Gates Glidden drills.[2]

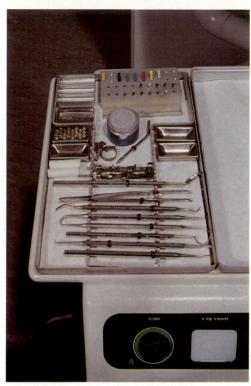

14.3   An endodontic instrument tray.

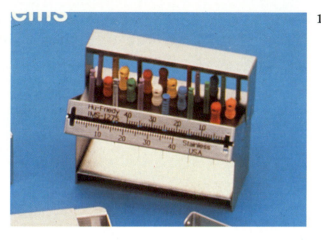

14.4   Other endodontic instrument holders are available.

The glass bead sterilisers

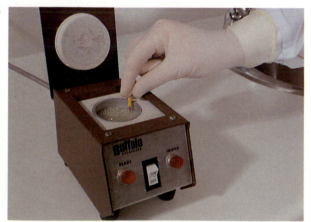

14.5   The glass bead steriliser.

During the treatment of multi-rooted teeth, glass bead sterilisers have been used to decontaminate files and drills (**14.5**). This may prevent the spread of infection from an infected to a non-infected canal.

After glass bead sterilisation, 50% of stainless-steel Gates Glidden drills were found to separate.[2]

One study found that endodontic reamers could be successfully sterilised in 5 seconds using a 'safe air' dental heater.[3]

Re-use of files and Gates Glidden drills

Discard size 1 and size 2 Gates Glidden drills, once colour changes, and especially corrosion, are noted.[2]

It has been suggested that size 10 endodontic files should be discarded after one appointment and size 15, 20, and 25 files discarded after two appointments.[4]

Disinfection of gutta percha points

GP points may be disinfected using a solution of sodium hypochlorite (1:5) for 5 minutes.[5]

Irrigation of root canals

Thorough irrigation of root canals with sodium hypochlorite solution is good endodontic practice and reduces contamination within root canals. Endodontic irrigation syringes should not be re-used.

References

[1]Morrison, S. W. and Brown, C. E. The effects of steam sterilization and usage on cutting efficiency of endodontic instruments. *J. Endodont.*, 1989;**15**:427–31.

[2]Zettlemoyer, T. L., Goeric, A. C., Nagy, W. W., Grabow, W. Effects of sterilization procedures on the cutting efficiency of stainless steel and carbon steel Gates Glidden drills. *J. Endodont.*, 1989;**15**:522–5.

[3]Forrester, N. and Douglas, C. W. I. Use of the 'safe air' dental heater for sterilizing endodontic reamers. *Br. Dent. J.*, 1988;**165**:290.

[4]Weine, F. S. *Endodontic Therapy*, 3rd edn., St. Louis, C. V. Mosby, 1982;266.

[5]Linke, H. A. B. and Chohayab, A. A. Effective surface sterilization of G.P. points. *Oral Surg.*, 1983;**55**:73–7.

15. Infection Control in Radiology

Dental radiographic equipment and dental radiographs may become contaminated with blood and saliva containing potentially pathogenic micro-organisms.

One study showed that *Streptococcus pyogenes, Staphylococcus aureus,* and *Streptococcus pneumoniae* may be transferred from one patient to another by contact with dental radiographic equipment and some micro-organisms were found to survive up to 48 hours on equipment surfaces.[1]

It has also been shown that radiographic films can transfer micro-organisms to darkroom equipment and that bacteria from radiographic film can survive processing.[2,3]

The aims of infection control in radiology are:

- To prevent contamination of radiographic equipment during radiography.
- To prevent contamination of radiographic film by patients.
- To prevent cross contamination from the film to the radiographic processing equipment.

Radiographic Equipment

Intra-oral X-ray equipment

The following surfaces should be either covered, or disinfected after use:

- X-ray cone (**15.1, 15.2**).
- X-ray tube head.
- Exposure controls and panel (**15.3, 15.4**).

Heat sterilise non-disposable film-holding devices using the autoclave or chemiclave.

The plastic wrap used to cover the dental X-ray machine KVp meter may possess a static charge which can deflect the meter needle, inducing erroneous KVp meter readings.[4] Dental X-ray machine operators should select meter readings prior to covering with plastic wrap. The initial settings should not be adjusted if the meter needle is later deflected by the presence of the wrap, as this may produce incorrect radiograph exposures.

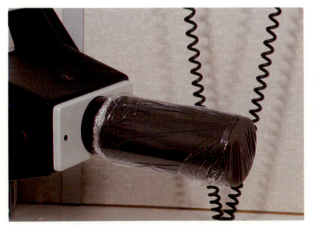

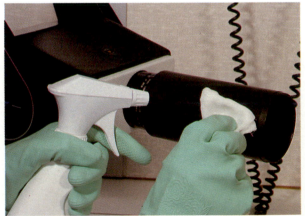

15.1 Cover X-ray cone.

15.2 Disinfect X-ray cone.

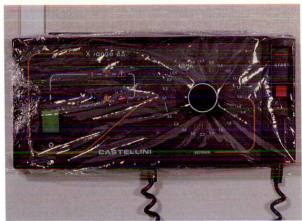

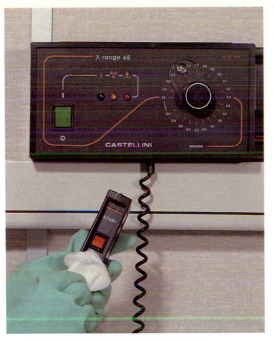

15.3 Cover exposure controls and panel.

15.4 Disinfect exposure controls and panel.

Panoramic equipment

Cover the following surfaces or disinfect after use:

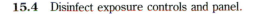

- Chin rest.
- Head positioner guides.
- Control panel and exposure button.
- Patient hand grips.

Heat-sterilise panoramic bite blocks using a chemi-clave or autoclave.

Disposable latex gloves should be worn when taking radiographs.

Contamination of Radiographs

Intra-oral radiographs become contaminated with saliva and possibly blood.

Plastic envelopes (**15.5 & 15.6**) or clingfilm may be used to protect intra-oral radiographs from contact with blood and saliva. The film envelope or cover is wiped and placed in an Environmental Protection Agency (EPA) approved disinfectant for 10 minutes, rinsed, and wiped dry (**15.7**). The film is then removed from the envelope prior to developing. This procedure minimises transfer of micro-organisms from intra-oral radiographs to the darkroom or processing equipment.

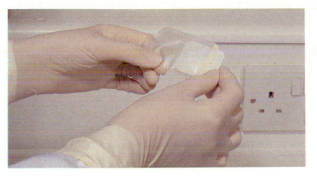

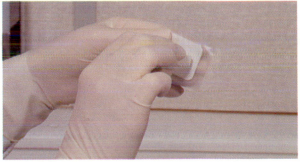

15.5 The radiograph is placed in the plastic envelope which is sealed.

15.6 The Kodak envelope with stick-on film holder.

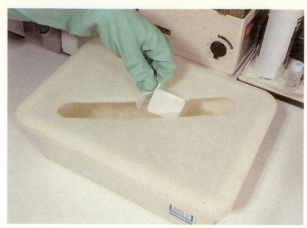

The film envelope is placed in EPA disinfectant.

The Darkroom and Radiographic Processing Equipment

15.8

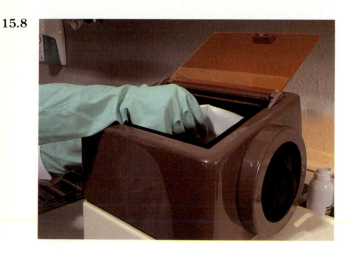

Disposable latex gloves should be worn in the darkroom when processing films in the darkroom, which have not been decontaminated, or when using a daylight loading processor.

The loading compartment and the film loading slots of daylight processors should be disinfected after use (**15.8**).

Darkroom surfaces and equipment exposed to contamination from films and handling should be disinfected:

- Counter tops.
- Shelves.
- Drawer handles.
- The process tank covers.

15.8 Disinfecting the film loading slots on the daylight processor.

References

[1]White, S. C. and Glaze, S. Interpatient microbiological contamination after dental radiographic examination. *J. Am. Dent. Assoc.,* 1978;**96:**801–2.

[2]Bachman, C. E., White, J. M., Goodis, H. E., Rosenquist, J. W. Bacterial adherence and contamination during radiographic processing. *Oral Surg. Oral Med. Oral Pathol.,* 1990;**70:**669–73.

[3] Katz, J. O., Geist, J. R., Molinari, J. A., Cottone, J. A. Potential for bacteria and mycotic growth in developer and fixer solution. *Dentomaxillofac. Radiol.* (Suppl.), 1988;**10:** 52–3.

[4]Jefferies, D., Morris, J., White, V. KVp meter errors induced by plastic wrap. *J. Dent. Hygiene,* 1991;**65(2):** 91–3.

16. Infection Control in Oral Surgery/ Implantology

Oral surgery and implantology procedures require additional infection control measures. Transmission of infection is more likely to occur, both to the dentist and to the patient, when undertaking extensive oral surgical procedures.

Everything used in oral surgery and implantology must be sterile.

Precautions to be taken include:

- Full surgical hand and lower arm wash is carried out before the procedure.
- Sterile disposable gowns, masks, and head covers should be worn in addition to eye protection (**16.1**). Gamma-irradiated packs, containing sterile operating kits, are now available (**16.2**) containing:
  - 2 gowns
  - 1 patient's drape
  - 2 surgeon's caps
  - 1 patient's head cap
  - 2 towels
  - 1 sharps container
  - 2 light handle covers
  - 2 module handle covers
  - 2 procedure trays
  - 1 roll of tape
  - 1 incineration bag
- Contamination of surrounding surfaces should be kept to a minimum:
  disposable paper or plastic covers should be used whenever possible on surfaces within the operating zone (**16.3**, **16.4**); hard surfaces within the operating zone should be carefully disinfected before and after the procedure; and strict aseptic technique, as described in Chapter 6, is essential.

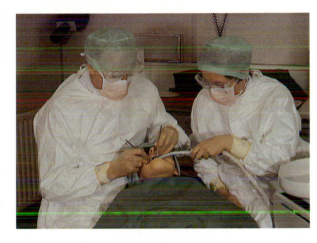

16.1

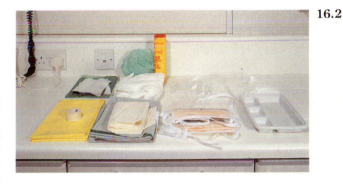

16.2

16.1 Gowns, masks, head covers, and eye protection during oral surgery.

16.2 Sterile operating kit.

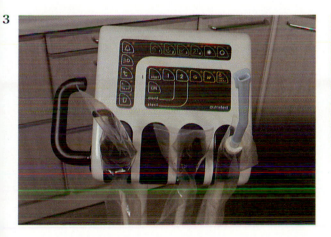

3

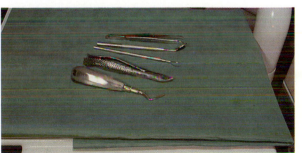

16.4

16.3 Make maximum use of covers to protect surfaces, e.g. plastic covers for aspirator tubes.

16.4 Sterile paper covers are available.

16.5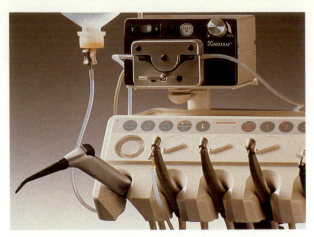

16.5 Saline solution supply. (Courtesy Siemens.)

- Use a pre-operative chlorhexidine 0.2% mouth-wash and swab the incision area with 0.2% chlor-hexidine before the incision.
- The irrigant or coolant solution must be sterile and uncontaminated with proteinaceous material found in tap water. Distilled, sterile water should be used. Some units have the facility to supply physiological saline solution, with separate hose feed to the instruments (**16.5**).
- After use, surgical instruments are immersed in a holding solution until they are ultrasonically cleaned. Care should be taken when handling and disposing of sharp instruments used, in oral surgery and implantology.

17. Illustrated Step-by-Step Procedures

Each dental office is different in design and equipment. The procedures described in this section are suggestions and should be modified to suit individual requirements.

Before undertaking the dental procedure

Dental assistant's duties

17.1

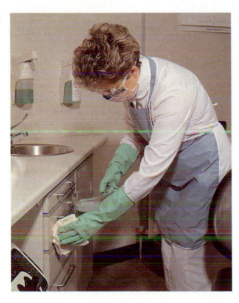

17.2

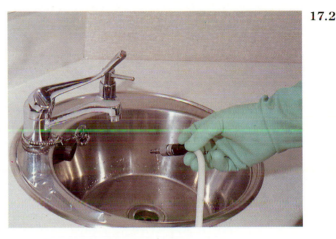

17.2 The turbine, air/water syringe, and ultrasonic scaler outlet tubes are flushed over a sink for two minutes. The water outlet supplying the mouthwash beaker should be run.

17.1 At the start of the day, the unit and cabinetry are cleaned using detergent and water.

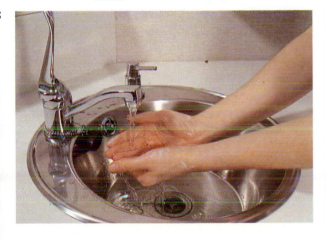

17.4

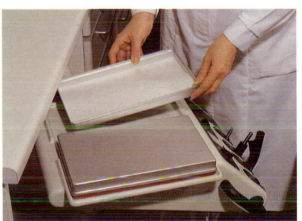

17.3 The dentist and nurse should perform a **full** hand wash.

17.4 All the loaded trays are placed in position:
Work and waste tray,
Nurse's tray,
Dentist's tray,
Anaesthetic tray,
Large, covered bur rack.

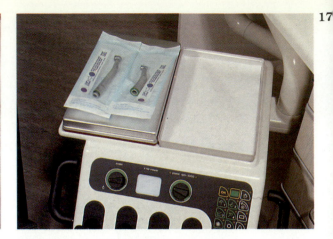

17.5 The holding solution is placed near the operating area.

17.6 The sterile, packaged handpieces are placed on the bracket table, and a preloaded mouthwash beaker is placed in position.

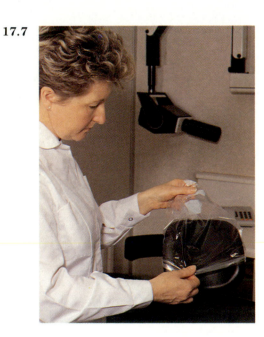

17.7 Equipment is covered as necessary.

Dentist's duties

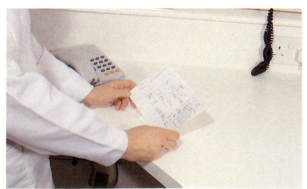

17.8 During this time, the dentist reads the clinical notes and radiographs and places them in a safe position where they can be seen but not touched or contaminated.

Dentist and dental assistant

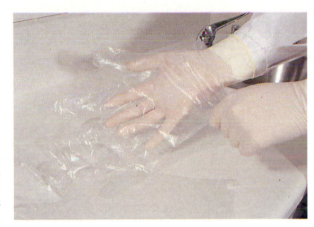

17.9 The dentist and DSA put on masks and protective eyewear, disinfect their hands with an alcohol-based hand-rub, and put on latex gloves. The **nurse** overgloves with low-cost polythene gloves.

Dental assistant's further duties

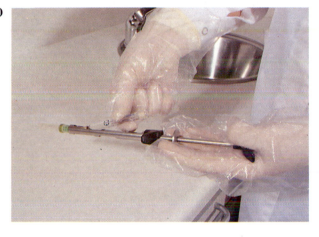

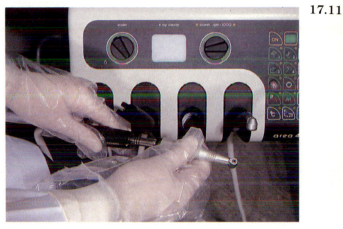

17.10 The sheathed needle and cartridge are fitted to the anaesthetic syringe.

17.11 The handpieces are fitted.

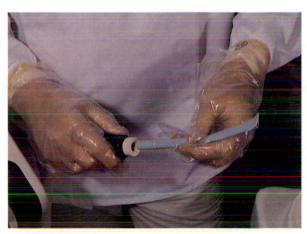

17.12 The lid is removed from the work tray and the air/water syringe, ultrasonic tip, vacuum suction tip, and saliva ejector are fitted.

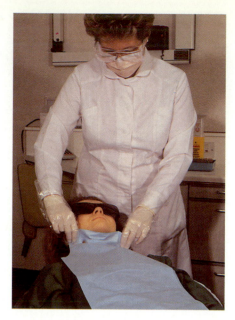

17.13 Disposable bib and protective glasses are put on the patient. If a composite colour shade is required, this should be taken now and the required shade of filling material obtained in a unit dose.

The dental assistant should remove the polythene overgloves and place them in a safe place, in case further use is necessary.

Procedures during dental treatment

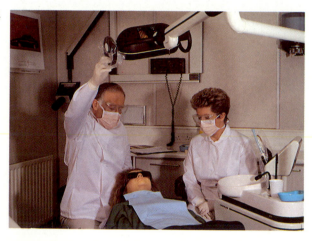

17.14 The light and chair are adjusted before the procedure is begun.

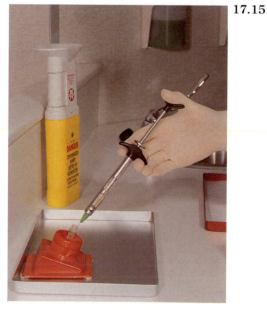

17.15 The dentist administers local anaesthetic and resheathes needle.

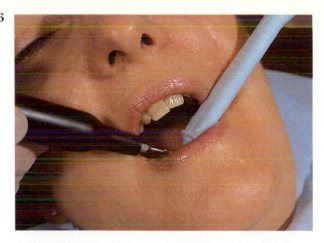

17.16 High-vacuum suction should be used when aerosols are created.

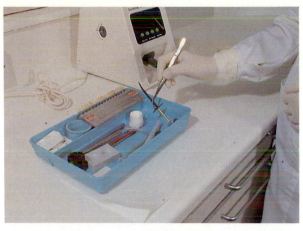

17.17 Sterile tweezers are used to take items from the nurse's and dentist's trays, and from the main bur rack.

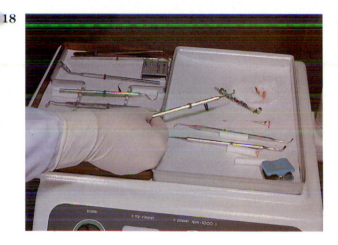

17.18 All used items are transferred to the waste tray.

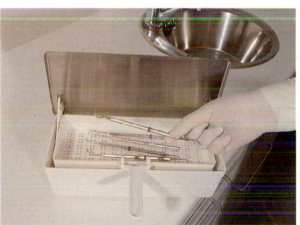

17.19 Contaminated instruments that are no longer required are transferred to the holding solution.

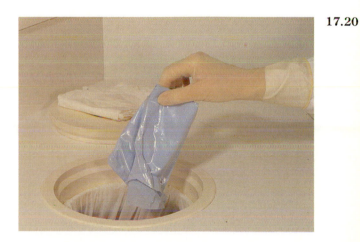

17.20 After the patient has left, the patient's disposable bib is carefully folded and disposed of.

Procedures after completion of dental treatment

Dentist

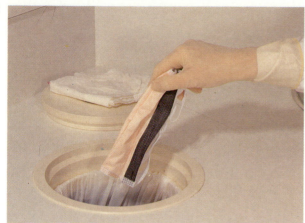

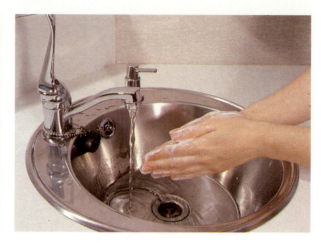

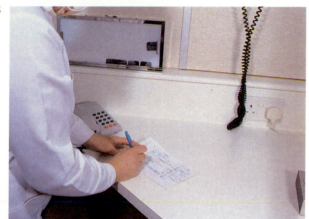

17.21   The dentist removes the mask and latex gloves, which are discarded, and the protective eyewear which is disinfected.

17.22   The dentist performs a hand wash.

17.23   The patient's notes are written up, outside the operating zone. These are taken straight to reception with the radiographs.

Dental surgery assistant

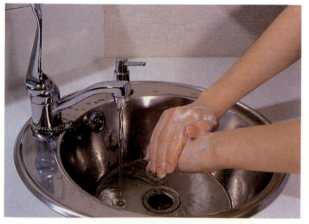

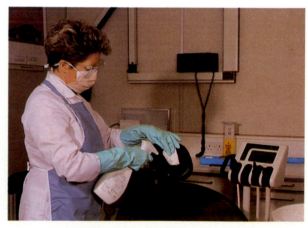

17.24   The assistant discards the operating gloves and performs a hand wash.

17.25   The assistant puts on utility gloves and plastic apron, and retains the mask and protective eyewear.

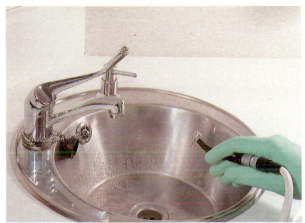

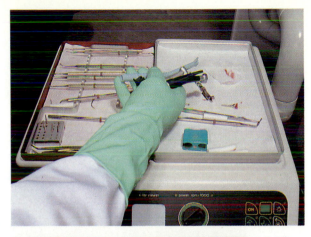

17.26 The handpiece, ultrasonic scaler, and air water syringe are flushed.

17.27 The vacuum suction tip, saliva ejector, handpieces, air/water syringe (or tip), and ultrasonic scaler (or tip) are removed and placed on the waste tray.

17.28 The anaesthetic needle and cartridge are placed in the sharps container located in the dentist's area.

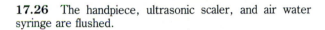

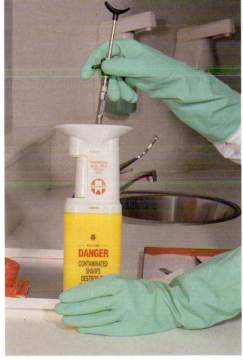

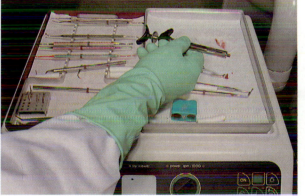

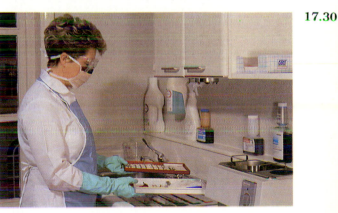

17.29 The unloaded anaesthetic syringe is transferred to the waste tray.

17.30 The waste and work trays are taken to the sterilisation area.

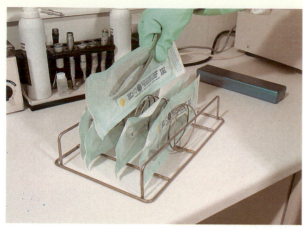

17.31 The holding solution is taken to the sterilisation area, disposables are discarded, and the handpieces and instruments are prepared for sterilisation. The waste tray is also sterilised.

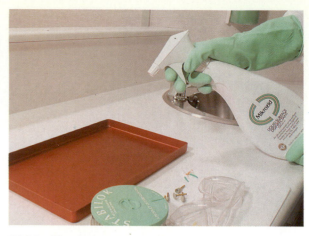

17.32 The remaining contents of the nurse's and dentist's trays are removed to a safe area using tweezers and the trays are disinfected.

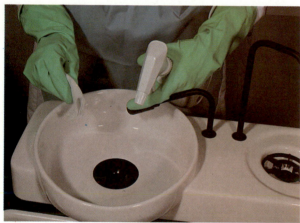

17.33 Contaminated, unprotected surfaces are cleaned and disinfected.

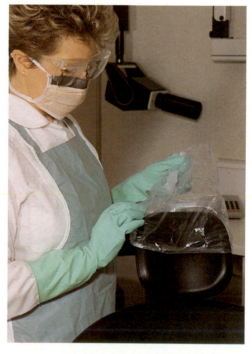

17.34 Protective covers are removed from certain surfaces.

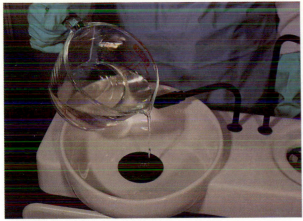

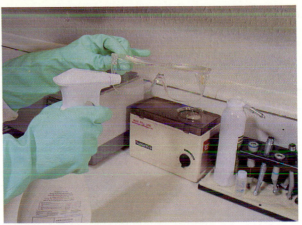

17.35 The spittoon drain is disinfected, and the waste filter is changed.

17.36 After all the instruments and trays have been placed in the autoclave, the dental assistant washes the utility gloves, removes and disinfects the protective goggles, and removes and discards the mask.

17.37 The utility gloves are rewashed, then disinfected and removed. The nurse performs a hand wash.

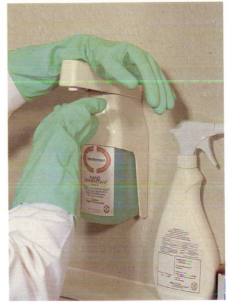

Additional routine at the end of the day

These are the duties of the dental assistant, who should wear utility gloves, mask, and protective eyewear.

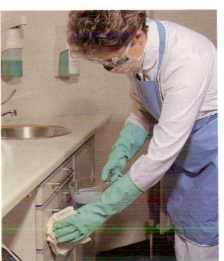

17.38 The dental unit cabinetry, sinks, and sterilising area are disinfected using an iodophor surface disinfectant.

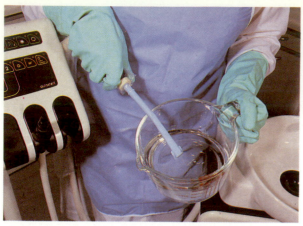

17.39 The high-velocity aspirator is disinfected.

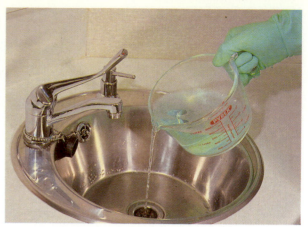

17.40 The sink and spittoon drains are disinfected.

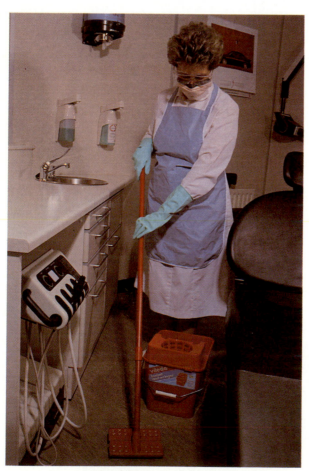

17.41 The surgery floor within the operating zone is cleaned and disinfected.

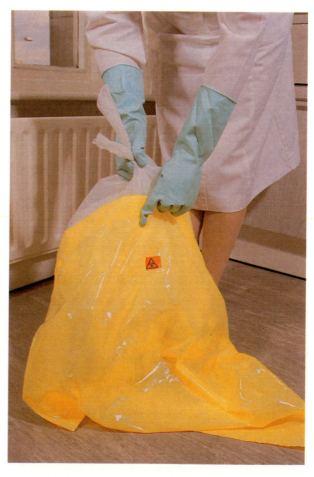

17.42 The bin liner is placed inside a heavy, outer bag, as described in Chapter 12.

18. Regulations and Guidelines

Guidelines: dental practitioners have a duty to their patients, staff, and themselves, to ensure that the procedures they use to prevent cross infection are adequate and in accordance with current *accepted* views and standards. Guidelines are procedures recommended by accepted bodies of dental opinion. Dental practitioners who do not implement relevant guidelines may be judged to be negligent and could be vulnerable if civil actions are brought against them by injured parties.

Regulations: are either backed by the force of law, e.g. OSHA regulations, or are promulgated by governing bodies, e.g. the General Dental Council in the UK. Non-compliance may result in fines or disciplinary measures being taken against dental practitioners.

USA: Guidelines

American Dental Association (ADA)

Dental practitioners should be familiar with and implement procedures described in the ADA guidelines.[1]

Centers for Disease Control (CDC)

The CDC is an agency of the Department of Health and Human Services (DHHS) and is responsible for the investigation and epidemiology of diseases that pose a possible threat to the health and welfare of the population of the USA.

Dental practitioners should be familiar with and implement procedures described in CDC guidelines.[2–6]

OSHA rely on the CDC for the accepted recommendations for health employers to follow, and therefore, the importance of these guidelines cannot be underestimated.

Note: At the present time, proposals have been presented to the American Senate to make the CDC guidelines on cross infection control *compulsory* with heavy fines for those found ignoring them.

USA: Regulations

Compliance with the following regulations is *essential*:

- Environmental Protection Agency (EPA) regulations.
- Occupational Safety and Health Administration (OSHA).
- State and local regulations.

Environmental Protection Agency

These regulations cover clinical waste disposal, labelling, and classification of chemicals, e.g. disinfectants. A working knowledge of these regulations is essential.

Occupational Safety and Health Administration (OSHA)

The OSHA was created within the Department of Labor (DOL). One of its objectives is to develop mandatory job safety and health standards and to enforce them effectively.

In September 1986, OSHA was petitioned by various unions representing healthcare employers' workers to develop a standard to protect workers from occupational exposure to bloodborne diseases.

On 19 October 1987 the Department of Health and the DHHS released a joint advisory notice entitled *Protection against occupational exposure to hepatitis B virus (HBV) and human immunodeficiency virus (HIV)*. This document contained the primary guidelines used by OSHA at present. Another updated and revised document was published in Autumn 1989. OSHA is in the process of developing a final health standard which should become effective in the near future.

At the time of publication however, OSHA has no standard that specifically addresses occupational exposure to bloodborne pathogens. There are a number of existing OSHA standards that provide protection for healthcare workers from these hazards, e.g. 29 CFR 1910 132 requires employers to provide employees with appropriate personal protective equipment. Section 5 (a) (i), the General Duty clause of the OSHA Act requires 'that each employer furnish to each of his employees employment and a place of employment that is free from recognised hazards'.

OSHA regulations apply to the dental healthcare setting and inspections are a real possibility.

General OSHA requirements: checklist

- Read and understand OSHA regulations.
- Follow CDC and ADA guidelines.
- Perform an exposure determination, i.e. classify tasks, work areas, and personnel in the dental office according to the degree of risk involved.
- Establish an infection control plan and maintain adequate written records of all protection procedures. This involves defining standard operating procedures for each task or classification which should include both the protective equipment and mandatory work practices necessary to prevent transmission of diseases.
- Provide a formal staff training programme in infection control.
- Know that, as an employer, you are responsible for the compliance of staff and, ultimately, the maintenance of their health.
- Understand and implement hazard communication regulations.

The written infection control programme

OSHA regulations on bloodborne pathogens require an employer to develop a written infection control plan. Such a written plan must contain the following information:

- Name of the employer.
- Name of the safety and health manager.
- Name of the programme co-ordinator.

The plan must state that the office is complying with OSHA instructions by:

- Performing exposure determinations.
- Providing HBV vaccination and post-exposure follow-up.
- Implementing an infection control programme.
- Providing a training programme.

OSHA requirements are based on CDC guidelines. Details of the relevant CDC and ADA guidelines must be written into the programme.

The specific infection control programme

Details of specific concepts and procedures required by OSHA must also be written into the programme.

- Universal precautions.
- Personal protective equipment, i.e. gloves, masks, eye protection facilities, and gowns.
- Infectious waste and sharps disposal.
- Housekeeping—cleaning and disinfecting surfaces.
- Labelling procedures (tags).
- Sterilisation and disinfection.
- Hand washing.
- HBV vaccination and post-exposure follow-up.

A model infection control plan which will satisfy the OSHA rule is provided in the ADA *Regulatory Compliance Manual*, which is available from the ADA (**18.1**).

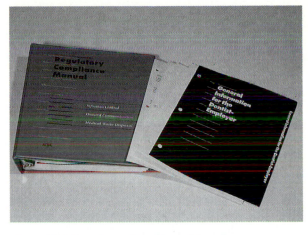

18.1

18.1   ADA Regulatory Compliance Manual.

The staff training programme

The OSHA rule specifies that a dental office must have a staff training and education programme, which is designed for and presented to all dental staff.

After receiving programme training, employees should be familiar with:

- The OSHA regulations.
- Categories I, II, and III tasks in the dental office.
- Epidemiology, modes of transmission, and prevention of HIV and HBV.
- Possible risks to the foetus from HIV and HBV.
- Location and proper use of personal protective equipment and their limitations.
- Proper work practices and universal procedures.
- Action required, and who to contact, if unplanned category I tasks are encountered.
- The meaning of colour codes, the biohazard symbol, and precautions to follow in handling contaminated articles or infectious waste.
- Procedures to be followed if a needlestick or other exposure occurs.

A *detailed* training programme is described in the ADA regulatory compliance manual.

A further training programme is provided by the ADA in a package of written materials and video tapes *Infection Control in the Dental Environment* (**18.2**). This is available from the ADA and is highly recommended.

The dentist or the safety and health manager must provide an acceptable and formal infection control programme. This should be in the form of lectures and administering examinations. Both the ADA compliance manual and the ADA training programme are designed for use in formulating and implementing such a formal programme.

Make sure new members of staff are properly trained in infection control procedures. Regular staff meetings should be arranged to provide updated information to all existing members of staff.

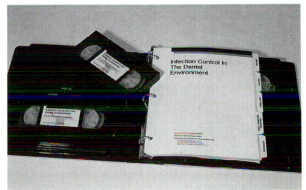

18.2

18.2   ADA Infection Control package.

Hazard communication regulations

OSHA enforce a federal regulation known as Hazard Communication Standard 29 CFR 1910 1200, on the rights of employees to know the potential dangers associated with chemicals which are defined by OSHA as hazardous.

Dentists must inform all employees of the dangers of hazardous chemicals used in the dental office and should train them to handle these substances safely. After training, employees must sign a training record and fill out comment forms. These records and files should be retained.

Many disinfectants used to implement cross infection control are classified as hazardous. Containers containing hazardous chemicals must be properly labelled. Disinfection trays containing liquids must be labelled with the information that is contained on the manufacturer's label, unless the solution is used immediately and then discarded. Spray bottles containing surface disinfectants must be labelled.

Material Data Safety sheets are supplied by dental manufacturers and suppliers of products that contain a hazardous chemical. A file of all such sheets must be made available to all employees and kept *up to date*.

A detailed Hazard Communication training programme is described in the ADA *Regulatory Compliance Manual* with sample record sheets and material safety data sheets. Two ADA advice sheets are also available.[7,8]

Medical waste disposal

Details of labelling and record keeping which relate to medical waste and sharps disposal are to be found in Chapter 12, and more information is provided by the ADA *Regulatory Compliance Manual*.

Buildings and equipment

An OSHA inspector will perform an inspection of the building and equipment, which includes eyewash facilities and waste receptacles.

Forms, notices, and record keeping

Keep careful records, to document compliance with the OSHA rule. This will provide defence against citations for non-compliance. All completed forms and records should be carefully filed and must be kept confidential. The following forms, notices, and records are essential:

- Poster 2203 must be displayed in a prominent position. A state poster may be required in certain states with OSHA plans.
- Exposure determination forms.
- Employees' medical records. Must be kept for 30 years and the employees must have access to their records.
- A written vaccination policy.
- Informed refusal form for hepatitis B vaccination.
- Written post-exposure and follow-up procedures: Exposure incident forms (OSHA form 200 and Supplemented form 101) are injury report forms which *must* be used in offices having eleven or more employees, and may be used in smaller offices. An employer who has eleven or more employees must post an annual summary of occupational illnesses. If five or more employees are injured in an exposure incident, a report must be sent to OSHA within 48 hours.
- Informed refusal by employee of post-exposure medical vaccination.
- Dates of implementation of each of the OSHA requirements, e.g. exposure determination, HBV vaccination, etc.
- Records and files relating to hazard communication regulations.
- Written infection control policy.
- Written training programme and training records.
- An employer must keep on file a copy of OSHA's *Access to Medical Records Standard*.

More details are provided in the ADA *Regulatory Compliance Manual* and sample forms are illustrated.

Complaints and inspections

There are two categories of OSHA inspection which concern dental practitioners: employee complaint inspections, which apply to any office; or programmed inspections, which apply to offices having eleven or more employees.

The most likely reason for OSHA to initiate an inspection would probably be due to a disgruntled employee. A dissatisfied patient, a new patient, or a patient of record who has acquired HBV or AIDS and who subsequently has been refused treatment by the dentist, may also file a complaint. Not only may OSHA be involved in this scenario, but municipal, state and/or federal statutes may have been violated which could leave the dentist open to a wide range of penalties, legal actions, and civil suits. External sources may be involved if the guidelines for management of material and infectious waste are not adhered to in the dental office. Reports of violation may come from sanitation services or cleaning services. This may not only cause OSHA to investigate but may also increase the possibility of local authorities and public health officials becoming involved.

The procedures followed by an OSHA compliance officer during either a complaint-generated or a programmed inspection are as follows:

- The compliance officer requests to see all relevant written files, records, and programmes, including poster 2203 (on employee rights).
- Following review of the records, the OSHA compliance officer interviews employees and inspects the dental office.

During an OSHA inspection, five areas of the dental office would be evaluated:

- Protective equipment, which should be 'provided, used, and maintained' properly.
- Contaminated waste.
- Biohazard tags.
- Housekeeping protocols: that all places of employment are kept 'clean and orderly and in sanitary condition'.
- General safety of the office: this requires that the employer must provide a safe environment for employees.

If a violation were to be found, the employers would be issued with a citation which would result in a fine. The citation letter contains an abatement date, which is the deadline by which recommended changes must be made and fines paid. The employer would be given 15 working days to respond to a citation.

The OSHA citation must be prominently displayed at or near the place of the alleged violation for 3 days or until the situation has been corrected, whichever is later, to warn employees of dangers that may exist there. The employer may: respond to a citation, requesting an informal conference with the OSHA representative; contest the citation; or comply with the recommended charges and pay possible fines. If an employer decides to comply, all changes must have taken place and fines must have been paid before the abatement date. Response to an inspection or a citation should be made only after seeking advice from the ADA and from a personal legal advisor.

Advice relating to OSHA inspections is provided in detail in the ADA *Regulatory Compliance Manual*.

In March 1991, OSHA initiated a new penalty structure which is outlined in detail in OSHA instruction CPL2 45B CH-2.

Voluntary activity

As well as providing penalties for violations, the Act also encourages efforts by workers and management to reduce workplace hazards voluntarily before an OSHA inspection, and to develop and improve safety and health programmes in all workplaces and industries. OSHA voluntary protection programmes recognise outstanding efforts of this nature. OSHA has published safety and health programme management guidelines to help employers to prevent or control employee exposure to workplace hazards. The local OSHA office can provide considerable help and advice on solving safety and health problems.

Consultation

Full assistance in the identification and correction of hazards and in the improvement of safety and health management is available to employers, without citation or penalty through OSHA-supported programmes in each state. These programmes are usually administered by the state labor or health department or a state university.

Important note

This section describes OSHA regulations at the time of publication. The final OSHA rule, which is soon to be passed by Congress, may differ from details described in this chapter. Dental healthcare workers should be familiar with such changes as they occur.

State and local (municipal) regulations

State and municipal regulations may have a greater impact on the dental practitioner, because the federal government traditionally delegates a number of powers such as the control of communicable diseases, to the state.

OSHA regulations may have been incorporated into state dental practice Acts or other state or municipal laws, which may have more serious consequences for non-compliance. The incorporation of OSHA regulations into state and municipal ordinances may result in suspension or revocation of a dentist's licence to practice if a violation is found.

Dental practitioners should understand and implement state and local regulations which are in force in their area. Dentists are advised to contact state dental boards and occupational and health agencies for information on specific infection control requirements in their state. State dental societies also have details of specific provisions of state laws.

UK: Guidelines

Dentists and their staff should implement the recommended standards of infection control described in the following publications:

British Dental Association Advisory Service. *The*

Control of Cross Infection in Dentistry, 1991.
Expert Advisory Group on Aids: *Guidance for Clinical Healthcare Workers: Protection Against Infection with HIV and Hepatitis Viruses*. London: HMSO 1990.

UK: Regulations

Dental practitioners must be aware of their legal responsibilities and specific regulations pertaining to infection control.

Health and Safety at Work Act, 1974

A dentist has a duty to take all measures that are reasonably practical, to ensure the health and safety of employees and other persons who use the practice premises. Failure to maintain the safety of equipment, or to adopt safe working practices, would expose a dentist to possible prosecution for a criminal act.

Where there are five or more people employed on the premises, a written statement of the employer's general policy with regard to health and safety must be brought to each employee's notice.

Practitioners can obtain valuable help on the preparation of their practice's health and safety policy statements from the guidance pamphlet C100 12/90, which is obtainable from local Health and Safety Executive (HSE) offices and from HMSO publications centres.

When patients are concerned about the cleanliness, hygiene, or lack of sterilisation in a dental practice, they frequently complain to the HSE or to the Family Health Services Authority (FHSA). The Health and Safety Inspectorate have powers of entry to investigate such complaints. Where serious risks to health and safety are identified, the inspectors may issue a prohibition notice, which takes immediate effect and remains in force until the corrective action has been carried out.

Where less severe risks are identified, an improvement notice may be issued, setting out recommendations on the time limits within which remedial action must be taken. In cases of serious breach of the Health and Safety requirements, or where a practitioner fails to respond to a notice, prosecution may ensue. There is however, a right of appeal where the facts are in dispute. The appeal must be lodged with an industrial tribunal within 21 days of the notice being issued.

Cross infection control is affected by the Health and Safety requirements in a wide variety of ways.

Autoclaves

Autoclaves are steam-generating pressure vessels, and as such are subject to obligatory safety inspections and certification at least once every 14 months. In the event of an accident occurring with an autoclave, e.g. should the door burst open, or a safety valve be projected across the room, the incident should be reported to the HSE, even if there are no injuries.

This can be done in the first instance by telephoning your local HSE Inspector, but should subsequently be put in writing, as detailed in the leaflet RIDDOR (Reporting Injuries, Diseases and Dangerous Occurrences Regulations 1985), which is available free of charge through the HSE.

Control of substances hazardous to health (COSHH)

On 1 October 1989, the general responsibility to ensure health and safety at work was extended, by the introduction of a subsidiary section of the Act. This lays down specific requirements, relating to the control of substances which are hazardous to health (COSHH).

It is encumbent upon a dentist to identify substances in the practice which represent a hazard, to assess the degree and nature of the risk, and to take action to minimise the dangers to those staff who handle them. Antiseptics and disinfectants are examples which relate to cross infection control. A more specific example is the use of glutaraldehyde, which can cause a variety of hazards. The COSHH regulations govern its labelling and storage, and give instructions for handling. These involve the wearing of domestic quality rubber gloves, protective clothing, and safety spectacles, all of which should be provided free of charge by the employer. The user must be familiar with the hazards and countermeasures and be aware of the correct strength of the solution, the purposes for which its use is appropriate, and the action which should be taken in the event of accidental spillage or contamination with the solution.

The HSE provides an excellent booklet describing how to carry out assessments of the risks, thereby saving a practitioner the expense of engaging outside expertise. The booklet may be obtained from HMSO Publications Centres by mail, or by telephone order on 071-873 9090. The address is PO Box 276, London SW8 5DT.

Other dental substances which are subject to COSHH include mercury, anaesthetic gases, methylmethacrylate, trichloracetic acid, and compounds containing iodine and phenol.

The regulations require employers to keep a record of injuries and accidents, including those which involve the use of substances hazardous to health. Where an employee suspects a health hazard at work, the first course of action should be to bring it to the notice of the employer or safety officer. If sources of specialist advice within the employer's organisation fail to resolve the problem the Employment Medical Advisory Service (EMAS) should be approached.

The Employment Medical Advisory Service

EMAS is an organisation of doctors and nurses who give advice on occupational health problems. It is part of the Field Operations Division of the HSE. EMAS has the same powers of investigation as HSE inspectors, but the greater part of its work is advisory in nature and is normally carried out with the voluntary co-operation of those who seek its help.

Initial contact with EMAS can be obtained through HSE information centres.

The General Dental Council

Guidelines which appertain to cross infection control have been laid down by the General Dental Council (GDC) and are to be found in Paragraph 23 of the red booklet *Professional Conduct and Fitness to Practise* issued by the GDC in 1989. This paragraph reads as follows:

'By the very nature of the work of a dentist, there has always existed the risk of cross infection in the dental surgery. Dentists have a duty to take appropriate precautions to protect their patients and their staff from that risk. The publicity surrounding the spread of HIV infection has served to highlight the precautions which dentists should already have been taking and which are now more important than ever. By following appropriate precautions to avoid cross infection, dentists may continue to treat uninfected members of the public with total security for all concerned as well as patients who might be HIV positive. Detailed guidance on the matter has been issued by the Health Departments and the British Dental Association. Failure to provide and use adequate sterilisation facilities may render a dentist liable to proceedings for misconduct.'

In those instances where a patient, colleague, or member of staff makes a complaint to the GDC regarding cross infection control, serious consequences may arise. Such complaints need to be made in the form of a Statutory Declaration made under oath, following which they will be considered in the first instance by the Preliminary Proceedings Committee. This committee may refer serious matters for consideration by the Professional Conduct Committee, and if, for the protection of members of the public it considers it necessary, may recommend interim suspension of a dental practitioner from the Register. There have been instances where practitioners who have failed to comply with the guidelines relating to cross infection control have subsequently had their names erased from the Dentists' Register.

National Health Service (General Dental Services) Regulations 1990

Allegations of failure to exercise adequate cross infection control are sometimes brought against dentists working under the General Dental Services as a result of a patient's complaint to a FHSA. In these circumstances, it is usual for the FHSA to seek an inspection of the practice premises through the agency of the Dental Reference Service. Unlike the HSE Inspectorate, Dental Reference Officers must give resonable notice of their intent to inspect a practice. A period of 2–3 weeks is a normal period of notification. Whereas HSE inspectors have a right of entry to all parts of the premises, Dental Reference Officers are restricted by the regulations to those areas where patients have access, for example, entrance halls, stairways, waiting areas, toilets and dental surgeries. With the agreement of the practice principal, they can also inspect staff quarters and dental laboratories. Where the FHSA receives adverse reports, these will be considered by the Chairman of the Dental Service Committee and if the reports are thought to reveal a serious problem, the practitioner may be referred for investigation by the Dental Service Committee.

Dental Reference Officers do not have the power to close dental practices, they can only make recommendations which must be acted on by the FHSA with whom the dentist is in contract.

The outcome of such investigations is usually to instruct the dentist to correct the problem which came to light, following which re-inspection is undertaken by the DRO to confirm that the premises are satisfactory. Under exceptional circumstances the practice will be closed during the period in which the remedial action is being undertaken.

Factors which commonly give rise to such investigations include complaints regarding dirty instruments, tarnished instruments, stained instrument trays, failure of dentists to wear gloves or not to be seen washing their hands, and the wearing of soiled protective clothing by dentists or their staff. The presence of torn floor covering, tears in the upholstery on dental chairs, or an unsatisfactory standard of decoration and general cleanliness are also likely to give rise to such complaints. Patients are increasingly aware of the importance of cross infection control measures because they now see them as being of life-threatening importance. It should be remembered that patients have a very different perspective of the surgery compared with those who work in it or whose responsibility it is to clean and maintain it. It is recommended that from time to time practitioners should view their surgeries from the same angle and positions as the surgeries are seen by their patients.

The Employer's Liability Act 1957

(Defective equipment) Act 1969.
(Defective premises) Act 1972.
Consumer Protection Act 1987.

These Acts are relevant because an occupier of premises has a duty to ensure that lawful visitors will be safe when using them. In the UK, under the Employer's Liability (Compulsory Insurance) Act of 1969, it is mandatory for employers to display a certificate showing they hold a current policy providing cover for damages which may arise in the event of accident, disease, or injury to any employee or lawful visitor to the practice.

If an injury were to occur as the result of a fault in the manufacture of equipment, the initial liability will fall on the employer who could then, in turn, recover indemnity from the equipment manufacturers.

The law relating to civil action

The law relating to civil action applies to measures for cross infection control in that a failure to maintain adequate control would leave a practitioner open to allegations of negligence.

Negligence can be defined as the failure to exercise reasonable skill and care. It may be the failure to do something that a reasonable person under given circumstances, would have been expected to do, or alternatively the act of doing something which a reasonable person would not have done.

A lack of knowledge of current regulations, guidelines, and procedures would not be a defence against an allegation of negligence.

In order for an allegation of negligence to be proved, it is necessary for a patient to show that the practitioner failed to take reasonable precautions which, under the circumstances, a body of reasonable practitioners would have observed and as a result of this failure that the patient occasioned harm.

There are time limits within which an action concerning allegations of negligence must be raised.

Adult patients and parents or guardians of minors should commence an action within three years of the incident, or within three years of the cause of the action first coming to their notice.

When a minor suffers a complaint and no action has been raised by the parent, guardian, or authority in charge, the time limit extends for three years following the attainment of the patient's majority.

The Limitation Act of 1975 does however allow for over-riding of these time limits in special circumstances and it should be noted that because a writ may be issued but remain unserved for up to twelve months, a practitioner may not become aware of an allegation of negligence for as long as four years rather than the three-year limit referred to above.

Where a failure of cross infection control is the result of an act or omission of a member of the practice staff, the employing dentist would be held responsible, i.e. hold vicarious responsibility, for the employee's action. This does not however absolve the employee from an individual responsibility for his or her own actions.

The disposal of clinical waste

Clinical waste has been defined as waste arising from medical, nursing, dental, veterinary, pharmaceutical, or similar practice, investigations, treatment, care, teaching, or research, which by nature of its toxic, infectious, or dangerous content may prove a hazard, or give offence unless previously rendered safe and inoffensive. Such waste includes human or animal tissue or secretions, drugs and medical products, swabs and dressings, instruments, or similar substances and materials.

Categories of clinical waste

Dentists are mainly concerned with the following categories of clinical waste:

Group A
- Soiled surgical dressings.
- Swabs and contaminated waste from treatment areas.
- Small quantities of human tissue (whether infected or not).

Group B
- Discarded syringes, needles, cartridges, sharps and broken glass.

Both of these groups usually require incineration, but occasionally special local arrangements permit supervised burial of such clinical waste at designated infill sites.

All waste contaminated with blood and saliva in association with dentistry must be considered to be potentially infected and needs to be disposed of in accordance with the Health and Safety guidelines.

Sharps

Sharps, which include needles, sharps, or blades and other sharp edged instruments, plus broken glassware which may have been contaminated with blood or infected body fluids, clearly need special attention in order to prevent infection of staff, cleaners, cleansing operators, and the public at large.

In 1988, the DHSS laid down standards for sharps disposal bins. The use of strong, puncture-resistant bins, which are secure and capable of incineration is now mandatory.

The containers should be clearly marked and provided with an aperture which, under normal conditions, prevents spillage or inhibits removal of the contents. Prior to disposal, they must be fully sealed and not more than two-thirds filled.

Prosecution of dentists has occurred where waste disposal operatives have suffered skin penetration, resulting from failure to comply with the correct procedures for disposal of sharps. Prosecution has also occurred, where clinical waste has been taken to public amenity waste disposal sites and left with domestic waste.

Additional categories of clinical waste include:

Group C

Laboratory and postmortem waste other than that included in Group A.

Group D

Pharmaceutical and chemical wastes. The disposal of mercury and waste amalgam also comes under this heading.

Segregation and disposal arrangements

The arrangements for segregation and disposal of clinical waste, form part of a general policy for health and safety and involve formal training of staff together with the designation of responsibility to a particular member of staff. Training of all personnel who deal with clinical waste, should include instruction in the following factors:

- Selection of appropriate colour-coded disposal bags.
- Training in the effective sealing of such bags.
- Instructions to handle the bags only by their necks.
- A knowledge of the procedure to be used following spillage of contaminated material.
- Instructions to check on the sealing of bags following their movement to a new site.
- The loose contents should never be tipped from one bag to another.
- Disposal bags should not be filled more than three-quarters full.
- Pressurised containers such as aerosols should not be placed in these bags, because they may explode on incineration.
- Clinical waste should only be transferred from site to site in specially designed vehicles.

Colour codes for bin liners and disposal bags

Light blue or transparent bags with light blue transcriptions

The contents of these should be autoclaved before disposal. These bags are specially designed to be steam penetrable and should be marked with autoclave tape so that it is clear whether or not the contents have been sterilised. Clinical waste from haemodialysis units is customarily disposed of in this way.

Yellow

All normal clinical waste designed for incineration should be placed in a yellow bag.

Yellow bag with a black band

These bags are for use where disposal by incineration is preferable but can be used where special arrangements have been made for disposal on land-fill sites.

Black

These bags are for normal household waste and should never be used for clinical waste.

Storage

Prior to collection, all bags containing clinical waste should be kept in a place where they are secure and cannot be interfered with by unauthorised persons, children, rodents, and insects. Ideally the site should be readily accessible to waste disposal operatives.

Leakage, seepage, and spillage

The accidental escape of contaminated material requires urgent action. It should be handled with heavy-duty gloves and any liquid spillage should be soaked up with absorbent paper towels or tissues. The contaminated area should then be gently soaked with a disinfectant solution and the room should be kept well ventilated. After soaking up the disinfectant solution with absorbent towels or napkins, the area should be cleaned again using water and detergent solutions, and finally dried.

A spillage of this nature should be recorded in an accident book, and the incident reported to the dentist in charge.

Local arrangements

Most FHSAs have come to negotiated local arrangements, through local dental committees and local medical committees, for clinical waste to be collected from surgery premises.

In other areas, arrangements have been made for dentists and doctors to take their clinical waste to certain designated collection points.

The use of these arrangements is not mandatory. Each practitioner is however responsible for disposal of clinical waste generated in his or her practice.

Strict controls over the disposal of sharps and clinical waste are defined by the Environmental Protection Act 1990, and dentists who fail to dispose of waste in an approved fashion may face fines of up to £20,000.

The Post Office Act (UK) 1969

There are certain restrictions on items that may be sent by mail. Laboratory items and instruments for repair (including handpieces) should be disinfected or sterilised before they leave the surgery.

Pathology specimens require special attention, and should be packaged to conform to requirements published in the Post Office Guide which may be obtained from main Post Offices and HMSO.

Only first class letter post and Datapost services may be used. The parcel post service may not be used. The outer cover or wrapping must be labelled 'pathological specimen—fragile with care'. The name and address of the sender should be written on the package, to enable contact in case of damage or leakage.

Section 23—Offences Against the Person Act 1861

Persons cannot be compelled to have a blood test against their will, or without their informed consent. To do so, constitutes an assault and battery.

The Venereal Disease Regulations 1974

These regulations control the dissemination of information about individual patients with venereal disease. Information provided by a patient should be treated in confidence. The regulations allow for the exchange of information between defined groups of healthcare workers, if it is to the benefit of the patient.

Dr David Rees, Dental Secretariat, Dental Protection, has kindly provided the information contained in the UK Regulations section.

The HIV-Positive Dental Healthcare Worker

UK

The GDC is of the view that dentists who know they are, or believe that they may be, HIV positive and who might jeopardise the well-being of their patients by failing to obtain appropriate medical advice, are behaving unethically and may be guilty of serious professional misconduct. It is the ethical responsibility of the dentist who believes he may have been infected with HIV to obtain medical advice, to submit to regular supervision if infected, and to cease practising dentistry if so advised. The GDC issued a statement to this effect on 13 January 1988.

The Expert Advisory Group on AIDS also issued recommendations relevant to dentists who know or suspect that they are infected with HIV.[9]

Infected staff are unlikely to transmit microbial agents to others if cross infection control measures are effective and this is not generally regarded as a reason for treating an HIV or other virus-infected job applicant or employee differently from others. This is discussed in a Department of Employment and Health and Safety Executive booklet, *Aids and Employment* (1986). Employees have statutory rights against unfair dismissal which are not reduced if the individual is infected.

USA

State dental practice Acts vary as to the limitation or restriction of practice for dentists who are HIV positive. Certain states expressly limit or prohibit practice, e.g. Washington, North Carolina, while other states limit the practice of the dentists with physical illnesses that threaten the patient or public health and safety, e.g. Texas, Virginia, and some states have no restrictions.

It is because health professionals are licensed by state agencies that these have the authority to issue regulations governing the practice of each health discipline. The regulations have the force of law, and violation of any regulation could result in suspension or revocation of a licence to practise.

Dental practitioners should be aware of state regulations which apply in their case.
Note: The first stage of a bill to make regular AIDS testing a mandatory requirement for all healthcare workers has been successfully introduced before the American Senate. If this becomes law, a HIV-positive healthcare worker would be prevented from treating patients.

The ADA Interim Policy, February 1991

'An HIV-infected dentist should refrain from performing invasive procedures or should disclose his/her sero-positive status.'

CDC recommendations—July 1991

Investigations of HIV and HBV transmissions from healthcare workers to patients, indicate that, when healthcare workers adhere to recommended infection control procedures, the risk of transmitting HBV from an infected healthcare worker to a patient is small, and the risk of transmitting HIV is likely to be even smaller. However, the likelihood of exposure of the patient to the healthcare worker's blood is greater for certain procedures, designated as exposure-prone. To minimise the risk of HIV or HBV transmission, the following measures are recommended:

- All healthcare workers should adhere to universal precautions, including the appropriate use of hand washing, protective barriers, and care in the use and disposal of needles and other sharp instruments. Healthcare workers who have exudative lesions or weeping dermatitis should refrain from all direct patient care and from handling patient-care equipment and devices used in performing invasive procedures, until the condition resolves. Healthcare workers should also comply with current guidelines for disinfection and sterilisation of re-usable devices used in invasive procedures.
- Currently available data provide no basis for recommendations to restrict the practice of healthcare workers infected with HIV or HBV who perform invasive procedures not identified as exposure-prone, provided the infected healthcare workers practise recommended surgical or dental techniques and comply with universal precautions and current recommendations for sterilisation/disinfection.
- Exposure-prone procedures should be identified by medical/surgical/dental organisations and institutions at which the procedures are performed.

- Healthcare workers who perform exposure-prone procedures should know their HIV antibody status. Healthcare workers who perform exposure-prone procedures and who do not have serological evidence of immunity to HBV from vaccination or previous infection, should know their IIBsAg status, and if this is positive, should also know their HBeAg status.
- Healthcare workers who are infected with HIV or HBV (and are HBeAg-positive) should *not* perform exposure-prone procedures *unless* they have sought counsel from an expert review panel, and have been advised under what circumstances, if any, they may continue to perform these procedures. Such circumstances would include notifying prospective patients of the healthcare worker's seropositivity before they undergo exposure-prone procedures.

The CDC have defined exposure-prone procedures as follows:

'Characteristics of exposure-prone procedures include digital palpation of a needle tip in a body cavity or the simultaneous presence of the HCW's fingers and a needle or other sharp instrument or object in a poorly visualized or highly confined anatomic site. Performance of exposure-prone procedures presents a recognized risk of percutaneous injury to the HCW and—if such injury occurs—the HCW's blood is likely to contact the patient's body cavity, subcutaneous tissues, and/or mucous membranes.'

At present, the ADA are in the process of defining their own interpretation of an exposure-prone procedure.

References

[1] Council on Materials, Instruments and Equipment, Council on Dental Practice, and Council on Dental Therapeutics. Infection control recommendations for the dental office and dental laboratory. *J. Am. Dent. Assoc.*, 1988;**116**: 214–8.

[2] Centers for Diseases Control. Guidelines for Prevention of transmission of human immunodeficiency virus and hepatitis B virus to healthcare and public safety workers. *MMWR*, 1989;**38**:5–6.

[3] Centers for Disease Control. Guidelines Universal Precautions for the prevention of transmission of human immunodeficiency virus, hepatitis B virus and other blood borne pathogens in healthcare settings. *MMWR* 1988; **37**:377–87.

[4] Centers for Disease Control. Recommendations for the prevention of HIV transmission in healthcare settings. *MMWR*, 1987;**36**:1s-18s.

[5] Centers for Disease Control. Recommended infection control practices for dentistry. *MMWR*, 1986;**35**:237–42.

[6] Centers for Disease Control. Recommendations for preventing transmission of human immunodeficiency virus and hepatitis B virus during exposure-prone invasive procedures. *MMWR*, 1991;**40**:1–9.

[7] Handle with Care. A hazards communication program for dentistry. *ADA News*, 1988; April 25th:9–12.

[8] Questions on chemical hazards answered. *ADA News*, 1988; September 19th: 24–6.

[9] The Expert Advisory Group on Aids. *AIDS: HIV Infected Healthcare Workers*. London: HMSO, 1988.

Index

—medical questionnaire 33–4
—needlestick injury 10
—oral signs and symptoms 17–19
—postexposure management 72
—risk areas 35
—risk groups 16, 34
—soft-tissue examination 35
Holding solutions 79, 115
Hospital disinfectants 99
Host susceptibility 9–10
Hot salt sterilisers 126
Human immunodeficiency virus *see* HIV
Hygiene, personal 53
Hyperhidrosis 42

I

Immunisation 37–9
—hepatitis B 20, 21, 38–9
—tuberculosis 22, 38
Immunosuppression 34
Implantology 175–6
Impression trays 162
—disposable 94–5
Impressions
—casting 164
—disinfection 159–62
IMS instrument cassettes 109–10
Infection
—control *see* Cross infection control
—sources 9–10
—transmission 9–12, 20
Infective dose, minimum 9
Influenza 38
Inhalation 9, 15
Injuries
—avoiding 68–73
—eye *see* Eye damage
—management 70–3
—needlestick 10
—*see also* Accidents
Inoculation
—hepatitis B virus 20
—transmission of micro-organisms 9, 15
Inspections
—Dental Reference Officers 194
—Health and Safety inspectorate 192
—OHSA 191
Instrument tray 78
Instruments
—arrangement and packaging 107–12
—contaminated 10, 75
—critical 30
—dishwasher cleaners 119
—endodontic 115, 116, 126, 169–71
—hand scrubbing 116
—non-critical 31, 157
—orthodontic 166–7
—rotary 115, 116, 126, 134
—semi-critical 30, 157
—sharp *see* Sharps
—sterilisation 113–35

—ultrasonic cleaning 114, 116–18, 167, 169
Intra-oral X-ray equipment 172–3
—radiograph holders 94–5
Iodine 47
Iodophors 87, 102
Irritant contact dermatitis (ICD) 42
Isopropyl alcohol 46, 47

J

Jeltrate Plus 161

K

Kaposi's sarcoma 18
Keratitis, herpetic 11, 24

L

Lamps 137
Latex gloves 55–61
—allergy 43, 44
—burns 60
Leukoplakia, hairy 17
Light curing units
—disinfection 85
—sterilisation 134
Light handles
—contamination 75
—covers 82–3
—disinfection 84
Liver disease 20–2
Lubricants, handpiece 130–1

M

Masks 11, 63–5
—anaesthetic 135
—contamination 64, 76
Medical history 33–4
Medical Waste Tracking Act (1988) 152, 154
Metal dentures 163
Micro-organisms 9–12
—hand skin 40
—inoculation 9, 15
Minimum infective dose 9
Mobile aspirators 91
Monitoring sterilisation 126–8
Mouthwash
—cup dispensers 80–1, 140
—cups 94
—pre-operative 176
—pre-treatment 90

N

Nails
—dentists' 11, 41
—herpetic whitlow 24
—paronychia 44
—psoriasis 45
National Health Service (General Dental Services)

Vinyl gloves 62
Virkon 88
Visors 66

W

Waste *see* Clinical waste
Waste haulers 153
Waste tray 79
Water retraction 128–9, 141
—test kit 144
Water supply, dental unit 144–7
Whitlow, herpetic 24

X

X-ray equipment 172–4
—radiograph holders 94–5
X-ray viewer 80–1

Z

Zinc oxide eugenol (ZOE) impressions 162

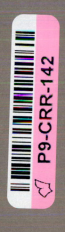

betty and rita go to paris

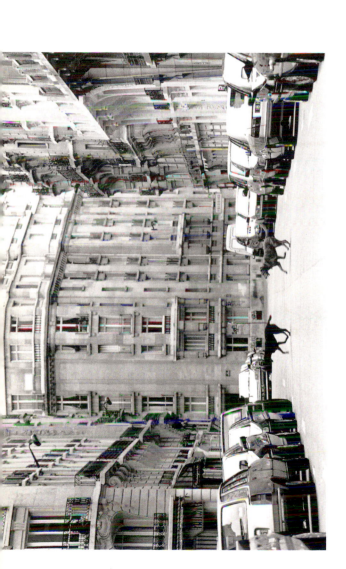

Text by Judith E. Hughes

Photographs by Michael Malyszko

CHRONICLE BOOKS
SAN FRANCISCO

Printed in Singapore.

ISBN 0-8118-2370-9

Library of Congress Cataloging-in-Publication Data available.

Book and cover design: Shawn Hazen
Cover photograph: Michael Malyszko

Distributed in Canada by
Raincoast Books
8680 Cambie Street
Vancouver, B.C. V6P 6M9

10 9 8 7 6 5 4 3 2

Chronicle Books
85 Second Street
San Francisco, California 94105

www.chroniclebooks.com

A special merci *to our bright and beautiful daughter, Maeve, without whose sublime adaptability to the new and challenging we could never even have considered a year abroad, and whose helpful hands and quick commands made all the difference to so many of these photographs.*

We're Betty and Rita, two traveling pups,
who took off for Paris and did the town up.

Our cab zipped us up les Champs-Élysées
where traffic was light that very first day.

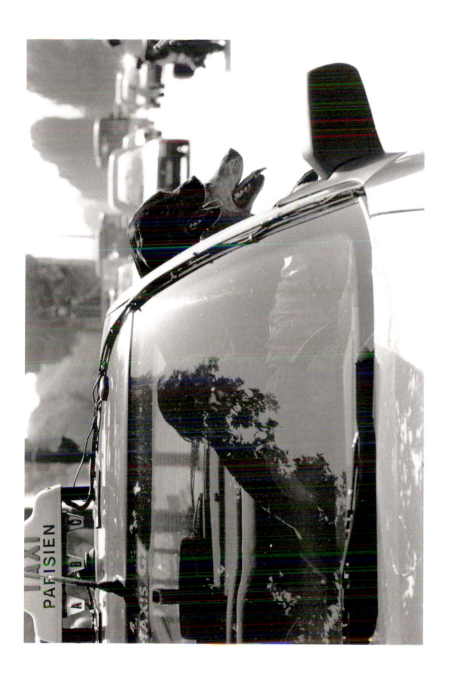

L'Arc de Triomphe was too big for this shot;
scrawny legs and plump bodies were all that we got!

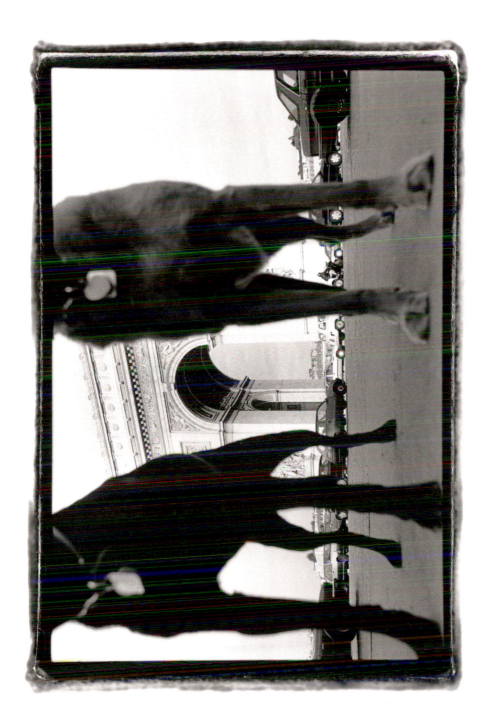

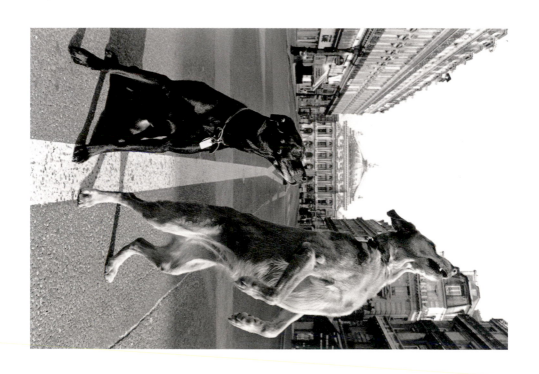

At the old Opéra—now just le ballet—
we gamely attempted a graceful plié.

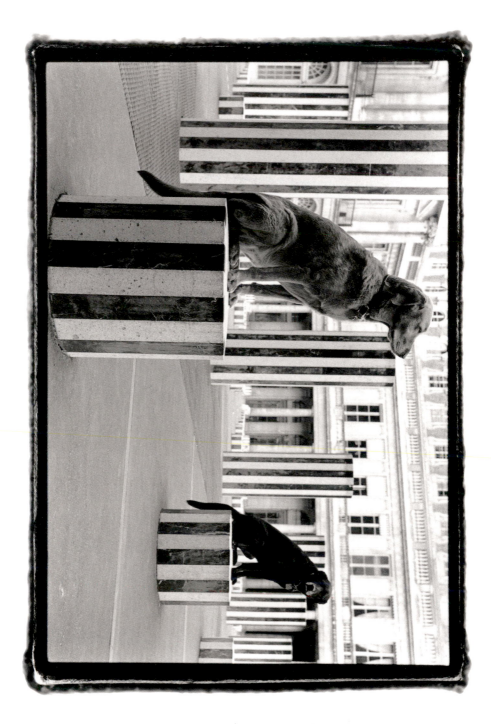

We got the mood right at

le Palais Royal

by climbing the posts and sitting up tall.

At Les Invalides we rolled with delight;

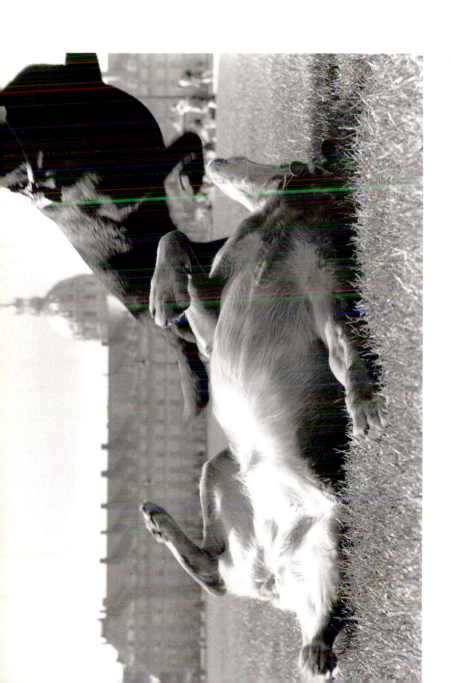

the Corsican's tomb was a beautiful sight.

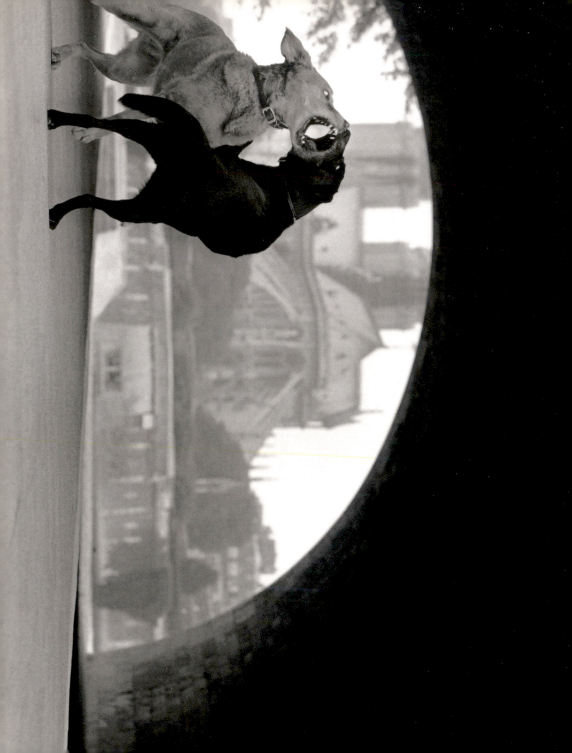

Then, being big dogs in need of some fun,

we saw Notre-Dame, but just on the run.

Three major musées were the second day's fare;

we took l'ascenseur instead of the stairs.

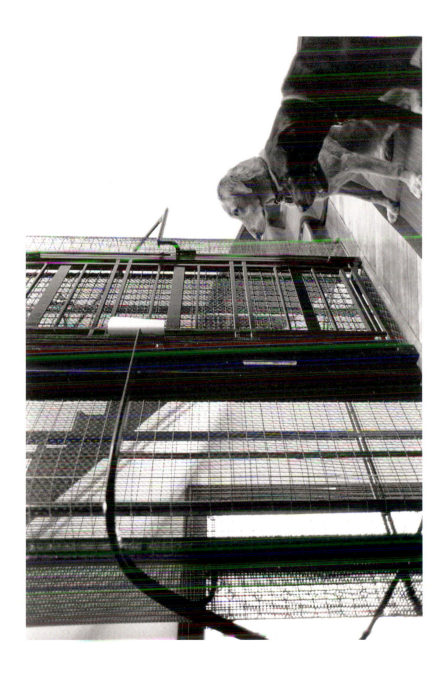

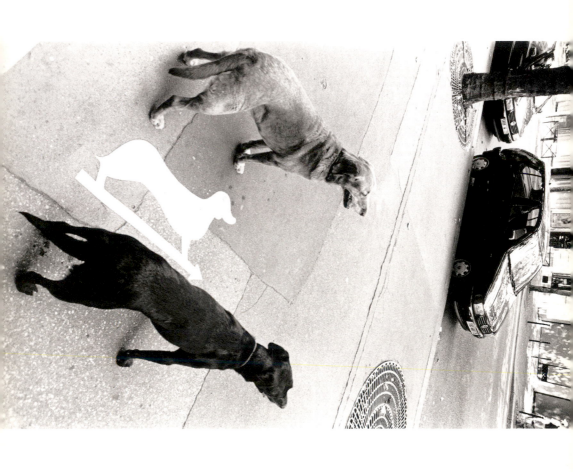

A strange illustration right on la rue

left nothing to chance on where to go poo.

Picasso's tableaux set our jaws all agape,

and we tried it right on with some paper and tape.

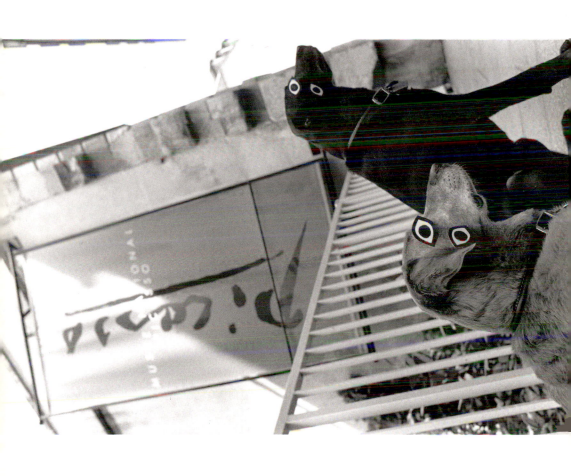

Le Centre Pompidou, across le Marais

looks built inside out and takes a full day.

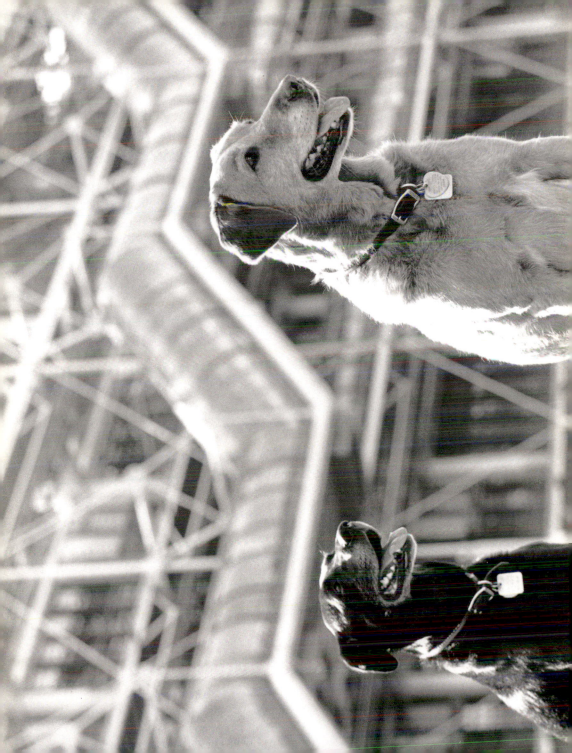

But hurrying through, we went on our way,

to make sure we'd have time to hit

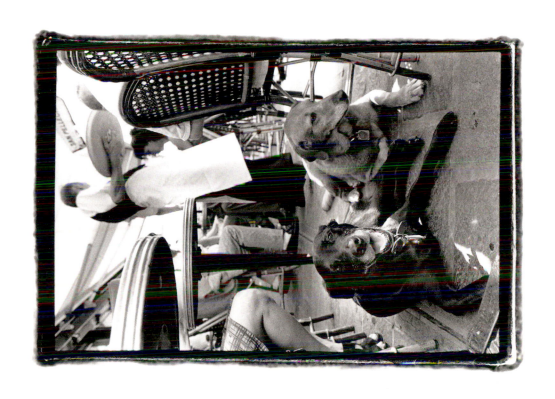

un café

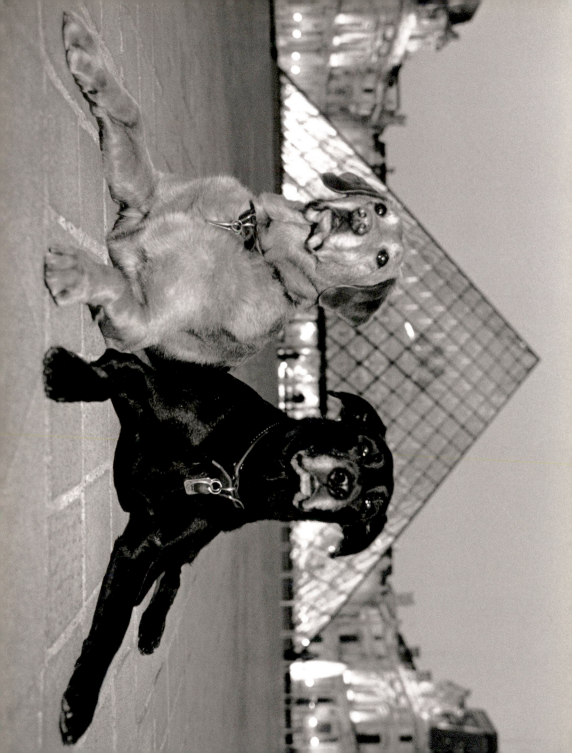

We ended our day au Louvre at sunset,

by the big pyramid—our best photo yet.

Day number three called for something quite new,

so from our balcon we took in the view.

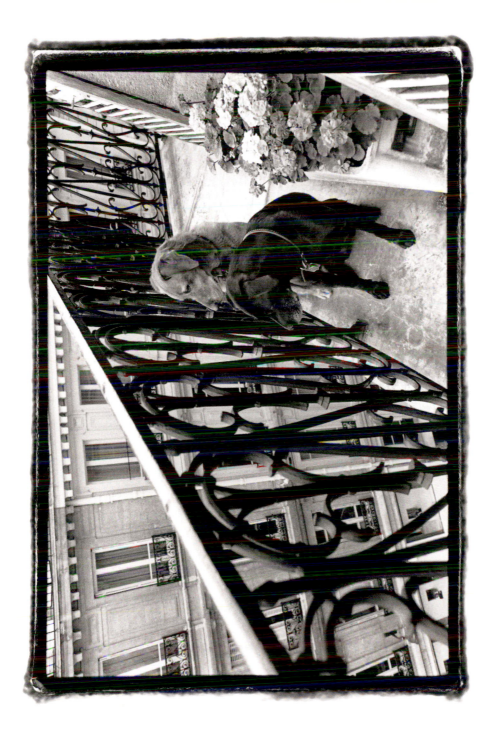

We opted to stay in our own quartier,
not even that hose could drive us away.

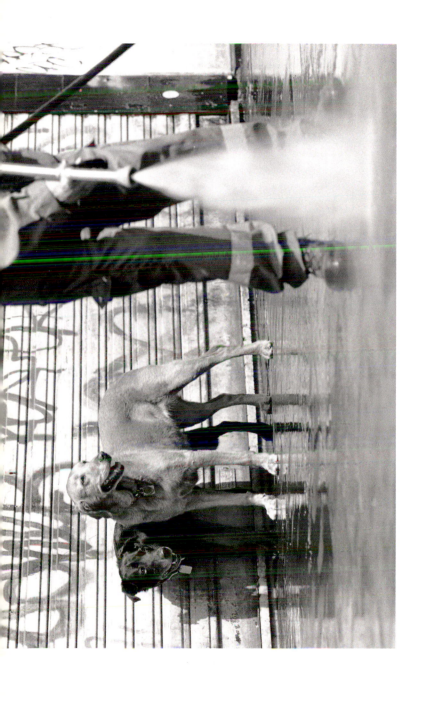

At last in the park once known as Les Halles

we met un caniche and soon had a pal.

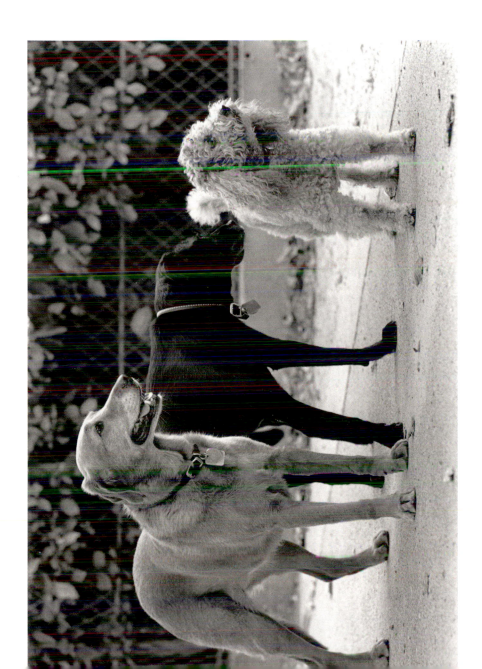

Under the plane trees the men played a game
by throwing a ball— pétanque was the name.

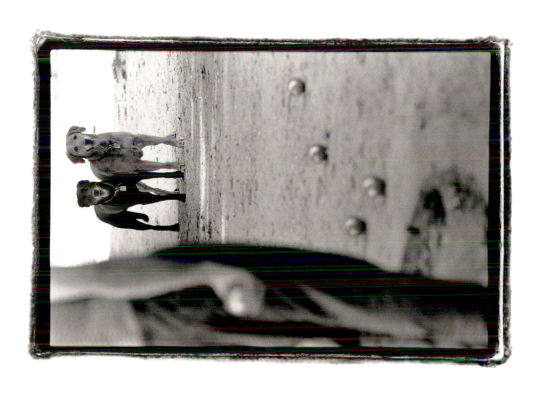

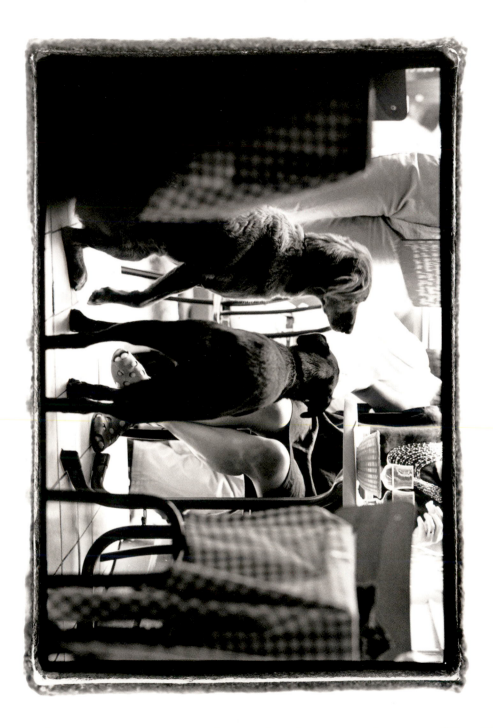

At a cute bistro politely we begged:

Please, just a morsel; it worked, we got fed!

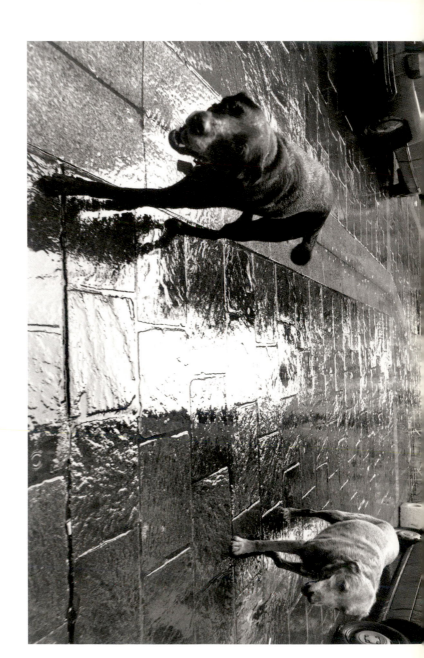

Then outside it rained and, soaked to the bone,

we headed chez nous and called the day done.

But sun the next day called for

un pique-nique

so we made up a list and raced off real quick.

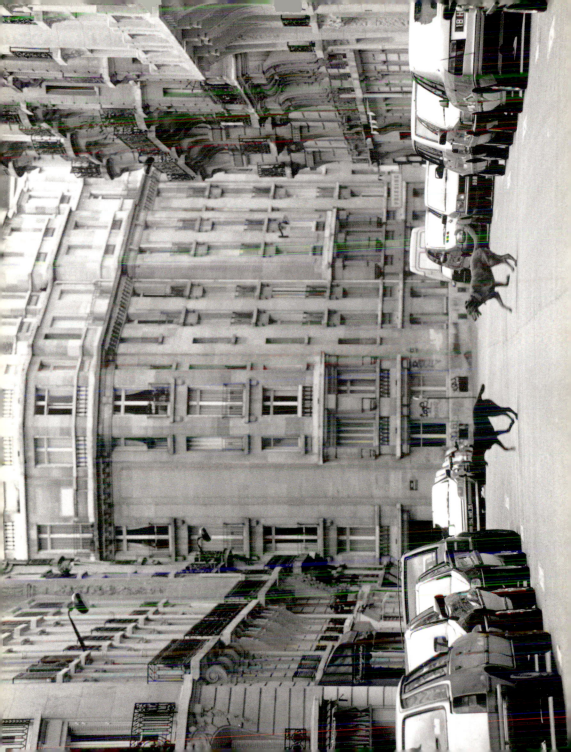

For meat, au boucher, where with one hungry look

we spied sweet saucissons up high on a hook.

42

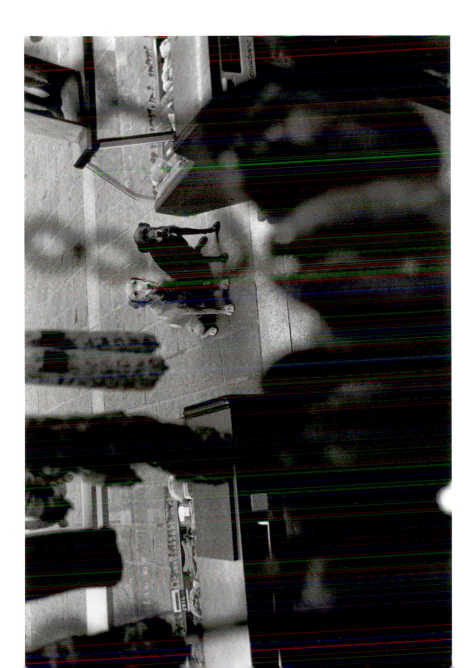

La boulangerie had lots of sweet treats,

but we bought une baguette

to go with our meat.

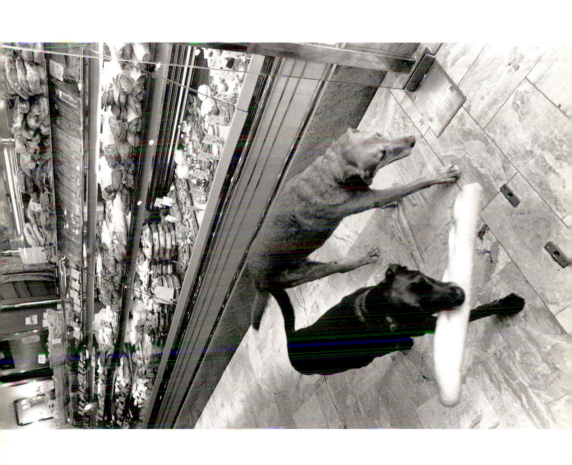

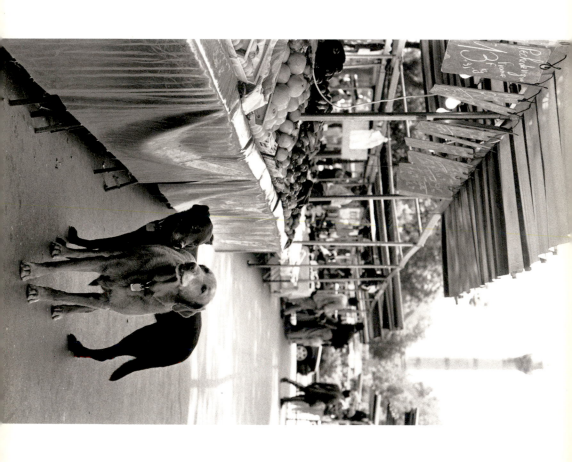

The open-air market out by la Bastille provided the fruit to round out our meal.

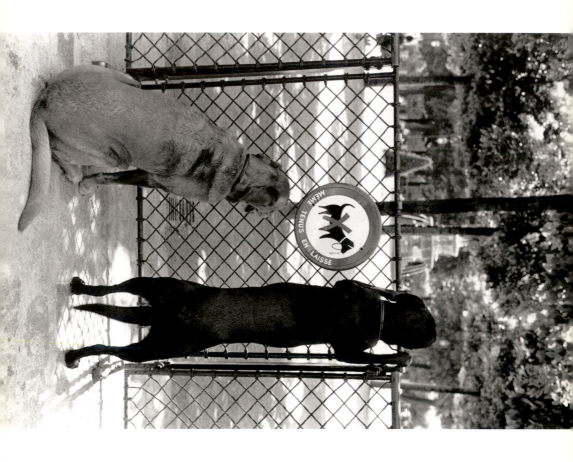

La Place des Vosges was green with no crowds,

but to our dismay we were not allowed.

49

Undaunted we crisscrossed la ville till we found

a spot with a view and plunked ourselves down.

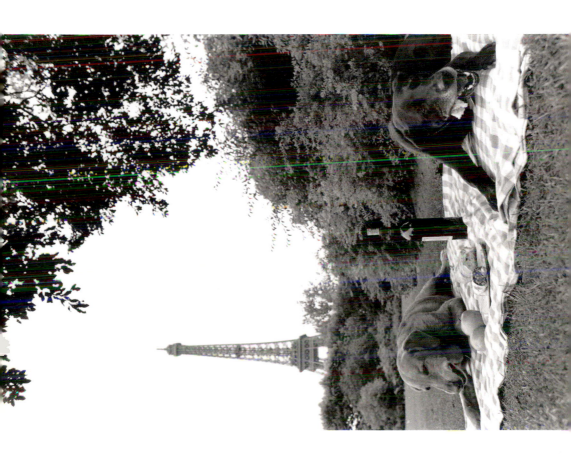

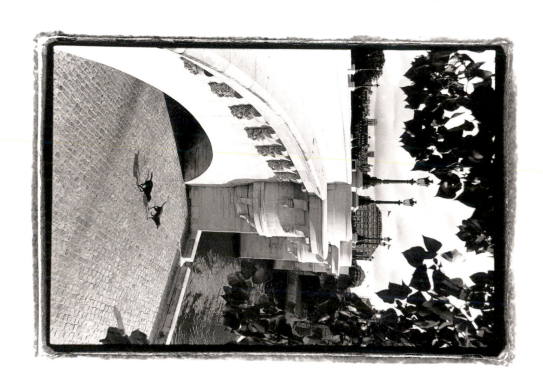

After all that, exercise was in order—

we ran by la Seine

and then hit the water.

A spot to cool off is what every dog needs,

so we dipped our paws at

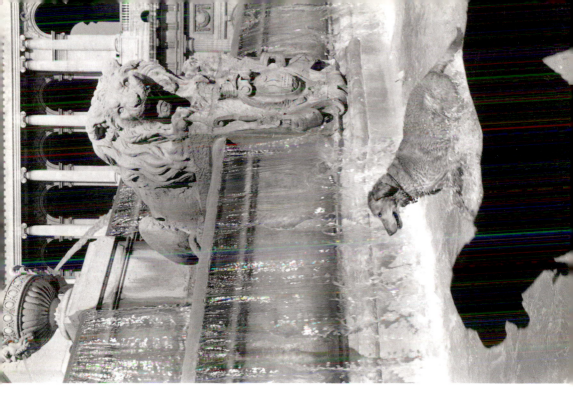

la Place St. Placide.

Big and refreshing and deep as a well,

but not so grand as la Place St. Michel

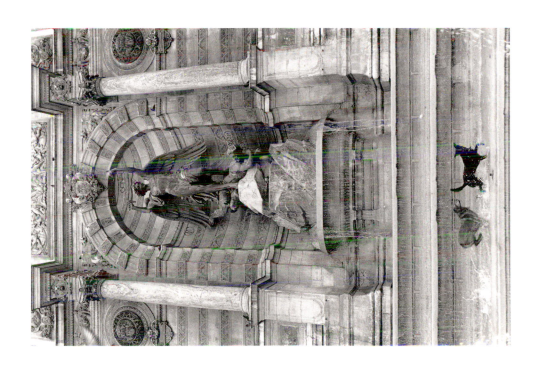

Back on the Right Bank we dove with panache

into the long pool by l'église St. Eustache.

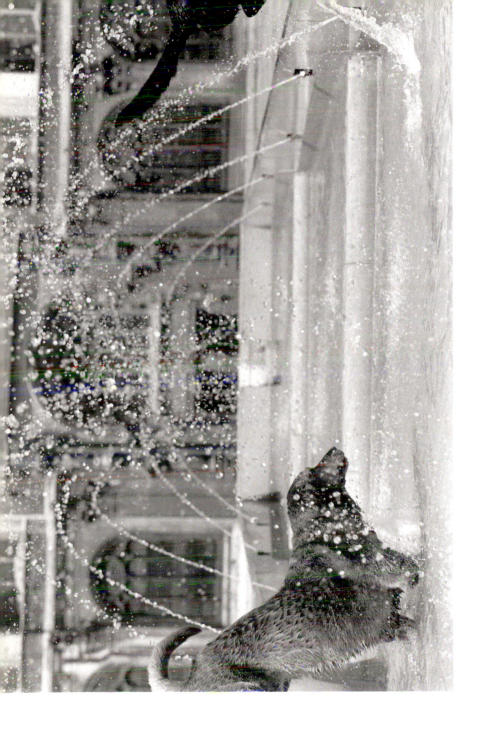

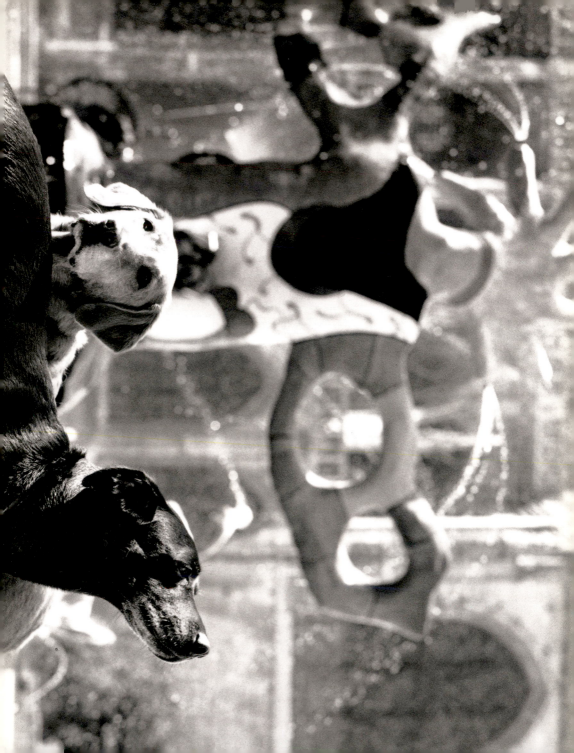

La Fontaine Stravinski

left us amazed,

entranced by the sculpture that moved as it sprayed!

At Père Lachaise we braved all the gloom

to pay our respects at Jim Morrison's tomb.

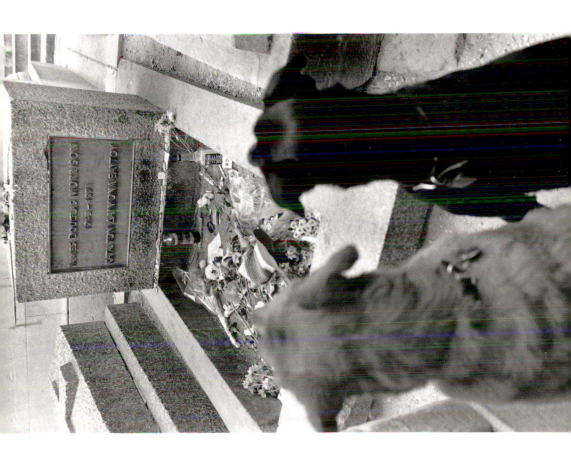

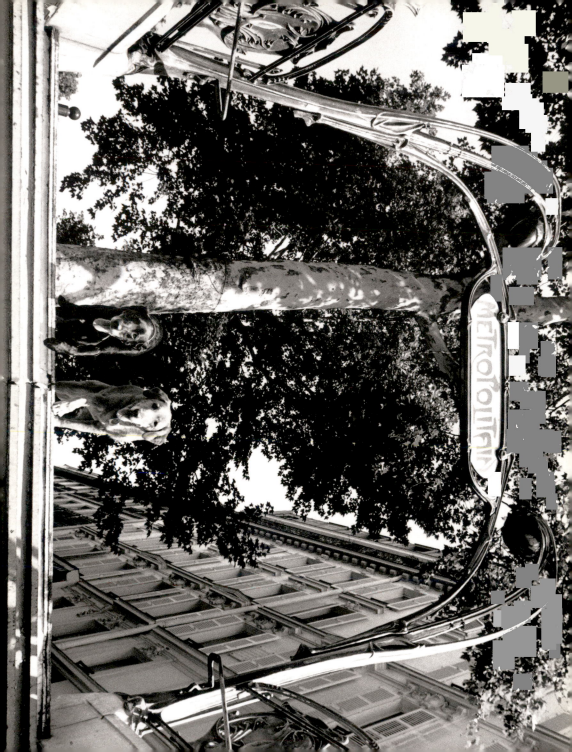

With so many places left yet to go,

on this, our last day, we tried le Métro

Back above ground au kiosque à journaux

we bought a newspaper to choose where to go.

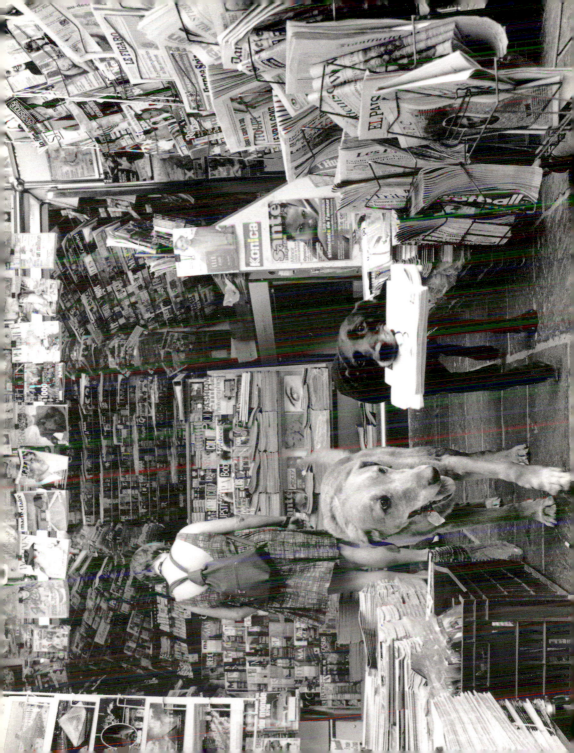

We wanted mementos that we could take back,

and les quais bouquinistes

had lots we could pack.

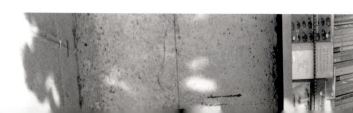
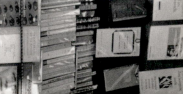

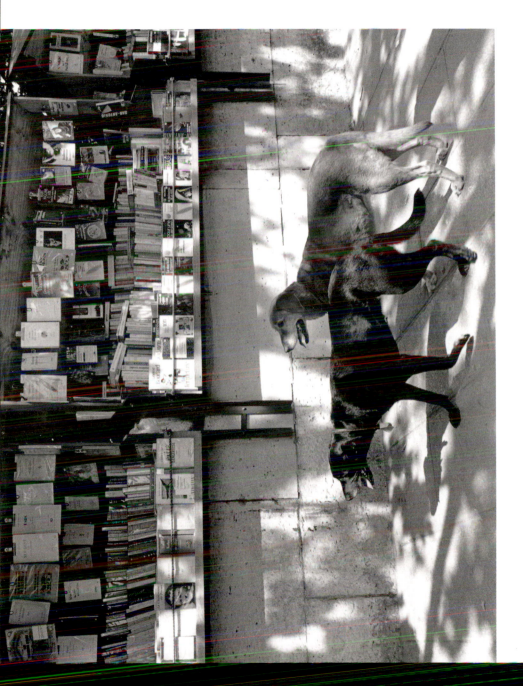

Au marché at Cité

we found the birds pretty

but locked in a cage. Oh dear, what a pity!

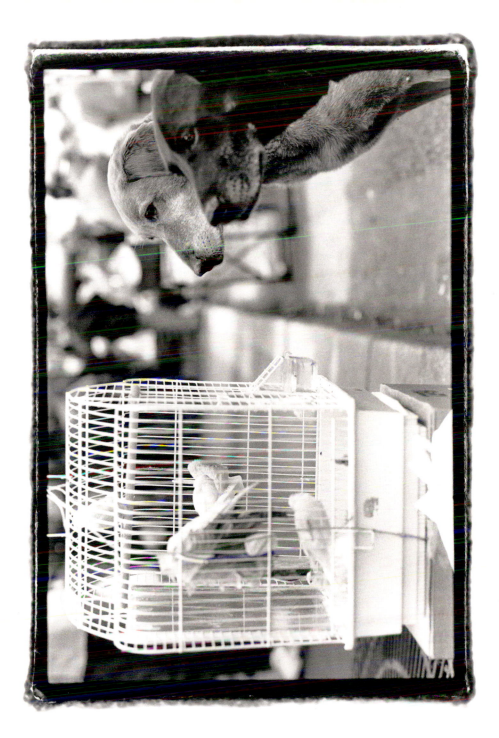

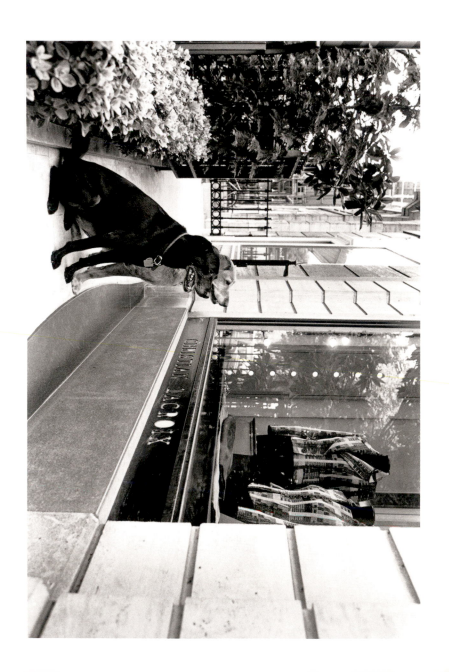

Back out in the Eighth, la mode caught our eye,

but the sizes were wrong, the prices too high.

73

Never defeated, we canines got smart
and sat for a portrait up at Montmartre

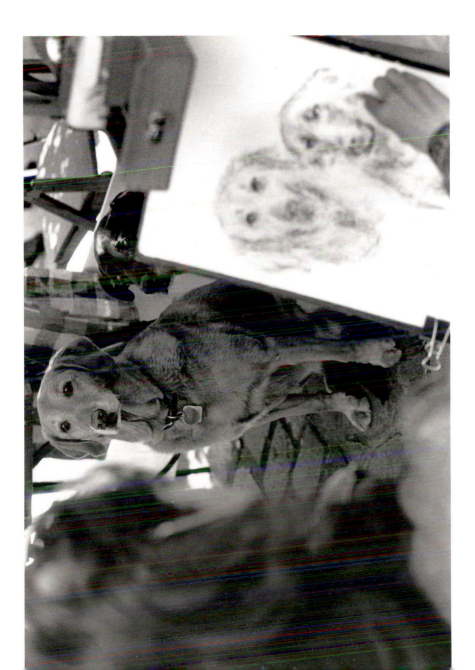

We said au revoir at our favorite café

and then headed out for one last soirée.

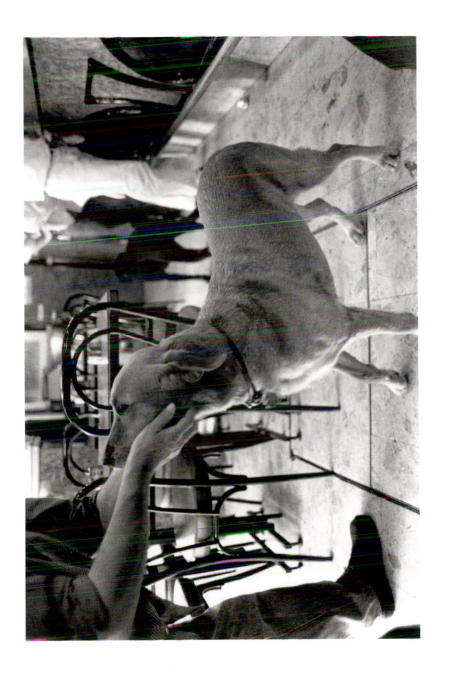

Le Moulin Rouge

should have been just the thing,

but it wouldn't be rocking in time for our fling.

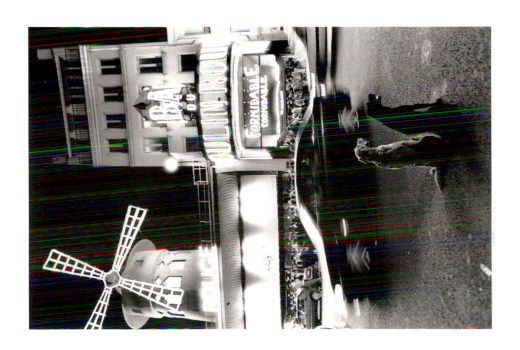

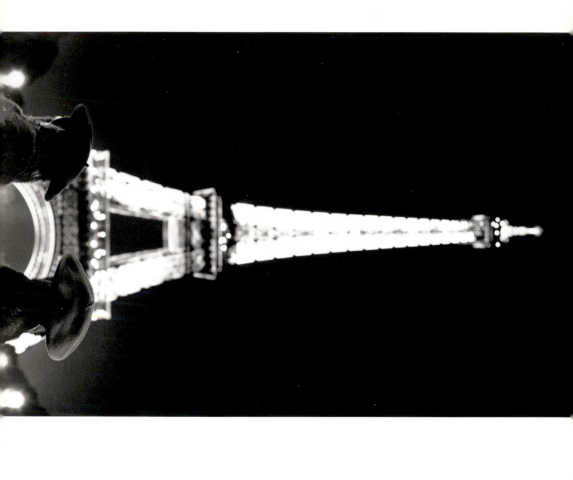

So, we raced off instead to that magical sight,

the famed Tour Eiffel all lit up at night.

afterword

Betty, born in April 1987, came into our lives almost immediately after the birth of our daughter. Betty is half golden retriever, half yellow lab, and all dog—sweet, loyal, protective, and utterly indiscriminate about what, when, why, and where she eats. Rita, born in August 1991, gained entry into the family because Judith provided Michael with an acceptable name for a second dog. She is half lab, half pitbull (we suspect), and all baby—a crooner, a total wimp, and a glutton for attention, having had the luxury of a big "sister," who fortu-nately got over her distaste for this competition after only twenty-four hours. The two have been inseparable ever since. To know them and see them wrapped around one another in sleep is to understand more deeply the yin and yang of life.

To say we all enjoyed making this book would be an understatement. When Michael would announce an outing by asking, "Are you ready to go to work?" the dogs would spring to life. (Of course, knowing canine hearing and language skills, they might have mistaken "work" for "walk," but it didn't matter, as they rose to each occasion to perform with enthusiasm.) The first photo we took was of the dogs looking wistfully into the entrance of the Place des Vosges; we knew we had a winner when a tourist stood behind Michael and took the same picture for her scrapbook! Photographing them in front of the Picasso Museum, we had fun noting the different reactions between tourists on their way in (quizzical) and those on their way out (hysterical)—clear evidence that museums can be both fun and educational.

Anyone who has ever been to Paris surely knows that the first response to a request of any kind is a polite but firm *non*. Anyone who has ever lived there knows that, whatever one is first told, with some patience and ingenuity it is possible to do almost anything. So when we decided to photograph Betty and Rita at Jim Morrison's grave, fully aware that dogs are not allowed into Père Lachaise cemetery, we went armed with previous shots in the series. When the guard approached, Michael flourished these examples, and she generously waved us on with a smile and a quick *"dépêchez-vous."*

Still, this book would not have been imaginable, much less possible, without the ever-present assistance and encouragement of the Parisians—the waiter who fed the dogs sugar cubes at the café, the baker who let us edge into her busy shop, the butcher who loaned us a ladder, the *vendeuses* at the *couturiers* who whistled and tapped the windows to attract the dogs' attention, and especially all our friends who supplied us with an endless stream of suggestions for the quintessential Parisian experience. Thank you, Paris, from the bottom of our hearts.

à bientôt